How to Survive the American High-Tech Diet

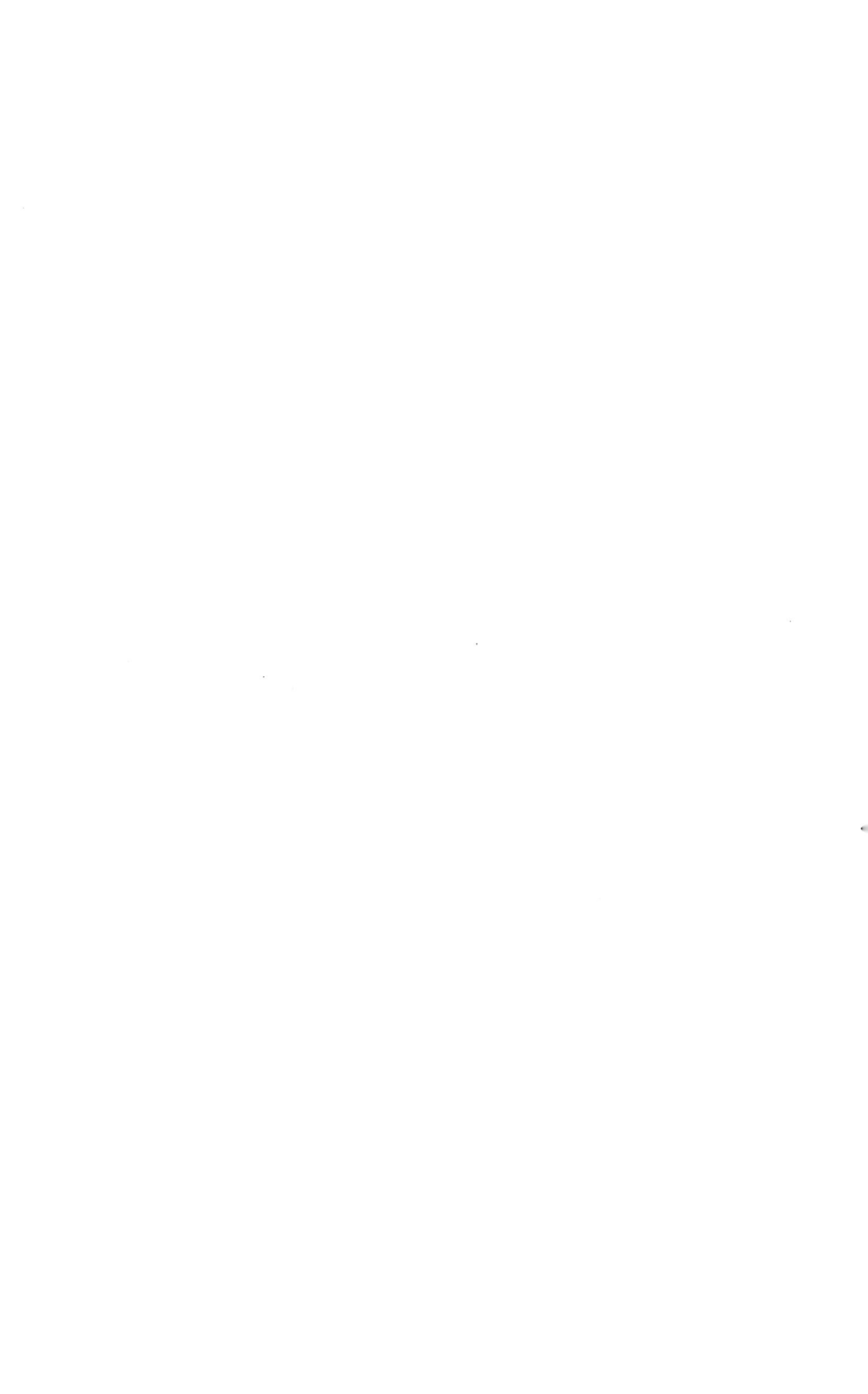

How to Survive the American High-Tech Diet

and Go From Toxic to Terrific

Workbook

Kathryn Parslow PhD, CCN
Certified Clinical Nutritionist

© 2017 Kathryn Parslow PhD, CCN
All rights reserved.

ISBN: 1974468976
ISBN 13: 9781974468973

Disclaimer

These videos, website and books do not provide medical or legal advice. They are for informational purposes only. Viewing them, receipt of information therein or the transmission of information from or to these videos/books/website does not constitute a patient-doctor relationship. The medical and/or nutritional information herein is not intended to be a substitute for professional medical advice, diagnosis or treatment. Always seek the advice of your physician or other qualified healthcare provider with any questions you have regarding a medical condition. Never disregard professional medical advice or delay seeking it because of something you have heard/read here. Use of this information constitutes acknowledgement and acceptance of these limitations and disclaimers.

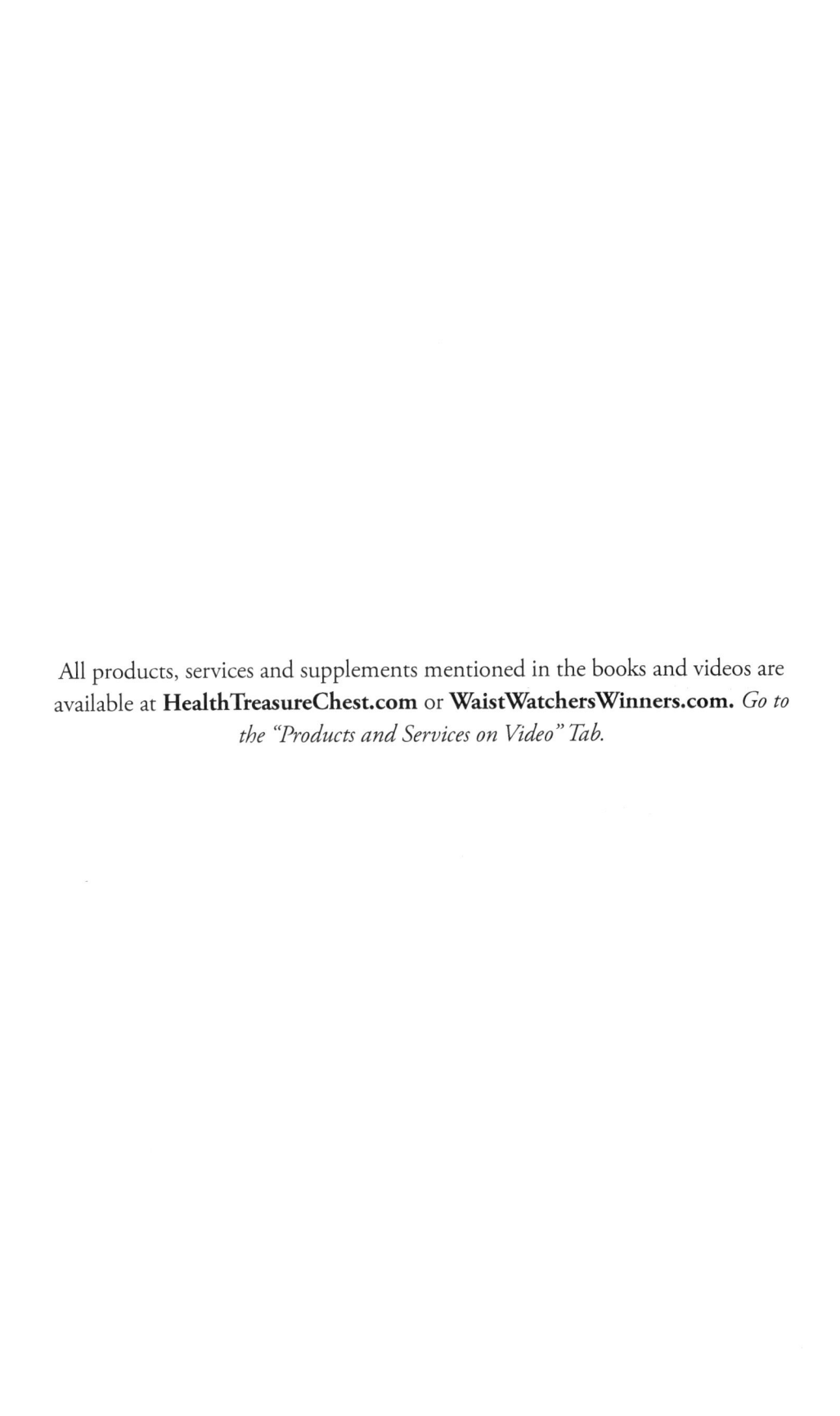

All products, services and supplements mentioned in the books and videos are available at **HealthTreasureChest.com** or **WaistWatchersWinners.com.** *Go to the "Products and Services on Video" Tab.*

Ladder of Achievement

⁂

I did
I can
I think I can
I might
I think I might
What is it?
I don't know how
I can't
I won't

⁂

Table of Contents

Disclaimer · v
Introduction · xiii

	Video #1 · 1
Topic #1	Blood Sugar – Crisis in America · · · · · · · · · · · · · · · · · · 3
Topic #2	Lifestyle Diseases – the One's We Cause · · · · · · · · · · · · 7
Topic #3	Digestion – Key to Health · 9
Topic #4	Inflammation – the Start of All Diseases · · · · · · · · · · · 11

	Video #2 · 13
Topic #1	The Bones · 15
Topic #2	Text Neck - 21St Century Ailment · · · · · · · · · · · · · · · · 18
Topic #3	Human Organs · 20
Topic #4	Exercising Against Gravity · 24

	Video #3 · 27
Topic #1	Healthy Eyes · 29
Topic #2	Healthy Skin · 31
Topic #3	The Brain · 32
Topic #4	WaistWatchersWinners.com · 33

	Video #4 · 41
Topic #1	Thinking Outside the Box · 43
Topic #2	What Have They Done to Our Food? · · · · · · · · · · · · · · 46
Topic #3	One Ingredient Foods · 50
Topic #4	Food Sensitivities · 52

	Video #5 ·55
Topic #1	Juicing for Life ·57
Topic #2	Sensational Smoothies ·59
Topic #3	Wheatgrass · 60
Topic #4	Sprouting for Mega-Health · · · · · · · · · · · · · · · · · ·61
Topic #5	Cell Phones ·62

	Video #6 ·65
Topic #1	The Children ·67
Topic #2	Food Deserts ·69
Topic #3	Problems with Processed Foods · · · · · · · · · · · · · ·73
Topic #4	Screen Time ·76

	Video #7 ·79
Topic #1	Fermenting ·81
Topic #2	Herbs ·83

	Video #8 ·89
Topic #1	Vital Vitamins ·91
Topic #2	Mighty Minerals ·95
Topic #3	Reading Your Body Like a Book · · · · · · · · · · · · · 97
Topic #4	Natural Cleaning Solutions · · · · · · · · · · · · · · · · ·101

	Video #9 ·103
Topic #1	Foods That Heal ·105
Topic #2	The Nutrition Researchers Who Went Before · · · · · · · · · · ·108

	Video #10 · 115
Topic #1	Detoxification ·117
Topic #2	How to Shop for Health · · · · · · · · · · · · · · · · · · ·120

Introduction

Recently, I wrote a book called, *How to Survive the American High-Tech Diet, and Go from Toxic to Terrific.* In the book, I relate many stories from my years as the nutrition educator and clinical nutritionist at the Tahoma Clinic, with world-renowned Jonathan Wright MD. There – I saw firsthand – the devastating effect the Standard American Diet (SAD) has on lives.

I realized that people genuinely needed survival techniques to protect themselves from their knives and forks. They needed to know that the "processed food industry" gives us artificial foods that are toxic and deadly, and that eating them – day after day and year after year – results in dire consequences.

As a nation, we are existing on the *foods of industry:* thousands of boxed, packaged, canned, shrink wrapped, fortified, dehydrated, salted, bottled, freeze dried, frozen and vacuum sealed foods. They've been artificially flavored, colored, sweetened, preserved, popped, puffed, crunched, crumbled, cracked, polished, bleached, zapped, emulsified, denatured, rolled and fried. Sprinkle in a whole host of pesticides and remove that annoying fiber. Just make sure the package is glitzy and tempting. It's all a recipe for disaster!

If a turn-of-the-century American were resurrected and thrust into a contemporary supermarket, they would be staggered by the enormous variety of available products – 10,000 or so instead of the 100 at his general store. Dazzling colors, transparent plastic wrappings, shiny metallic packaging and eye popping labels might make them think they'd entered the Garden of Eden.

Unfortunately, it's easy to confuse our seductively advertised lavish quantities of foodstuff with true nutritional riches. The fact is, most of our highly fabricated and cleverly packaged foods are compounded from a modest number of basic ingredients – the 100 or so relied upon by our ancestors. Yet, many of those 100 basic ingredients have been so altered by modern science, that the body does not recognize them as nutrients.

In the movie, *Super-Size Me,* a diabetic, hypertensive and overweight man is interviewed prior to a gastric bypass. "I suddenly went blind at work and my wife had to come get me," he said. "I drink *two gallons* of soda every day – and sometimes more." "Fifty-two liters every two weeks is what we buy," his wife said.

This equates to about 4½ cups of sugar a day, just in his drinks! What was most curious was their matter-of-fact attitudes. Not ashamed. Not defiant. Not challenging. Just completely oblivious that there were any consequences to their reckless dietary habits.

The doctor explained that the only procedure that really cures diabetes is obesity surgery. I thought, really? A procedure? What about a major dietary alteration to stop ingesting that much sugar in the first place? You'll read and hear other similar stories in these lessons and on the videos, including one by Phillip who had very similar experiences to our gentleman above.

Frequently, I walk the "climate controlled" mall in my town and am alarmed at the number of people who are morbidly obese. Morbid obesity means a person is 100 pounds over their ideal weight, or has a BMI (Body mass index) of 40 or more. BMI is how much of your body mass is "fat".

It begs the question; *how did we get here?* Is it too much sugar? Too many triple cheese burgers with bacon? Too much boxed, packaged and processed food? Too much screen time? Or is it too little natural, whole food? Too little movement? Not enough fresh produce? Or maybe it's just too much and too little of *everything.*

So, the more important question is, *what can we do about it?* Attempting to answer this question is why I produced the ten videos you will view, and the accompanying workbook.

Yet, there is hope. If we'll forsake the dietary recklessness which seems to have become a national habit, then we can get better as individuals and as a nation. But how? The key is taking that first step, figuratively and literally. This video series and workbook are dedicated to helping you learn how to take that step.

Your Mentor on the Journey,
Kathryn Parslow
drkathrynparslow@gmail.com

Video #1

Topic #1

BLOOD SUGAR – CRISIS IN AMERICA

In the first video, we discussed Phillip's case of severe blood sugar problems. No one had ever told him to avoid sugar. He loved sweet things, indulging in them all day long. And he was sick!

Thinking that a naturally-oriented doctor might find the cause of his seizures, he came to see Jonathan Wright MD at the Tahoma Clinic where I was the clinical nutritionist. Just getting him off all that sugar restored his health, stopped his seizures, and he returned to work in a few days.

At the clinic, I saw a plethora of patients with blood sugar problems. Jason described his wife like this: "When the toast pops up, she jumps. She spends two minutes deciding whether to use butter or jam. She gets mean, then sweet, then cries."

The Blood Sugar Diseases

Call it insulin resistance or diabetes or hypoglycemia or hyperglycemia. All these conditions are responses to how your body handles sugar. If you have type 2 diabetes or if you're at risk for it, extremely high blood sugar can lead to a potentially deadly condition in which your body can't process sugar or refined carbohydrates like white bread, cookies, cake and the like. Really, the key in all these "blood sugar" conditions is to stop eating all the sweet and refined junk.

Sugar Consumption in America and Obesity

Entire industries have grown around America's weight problems. But have the diet programs, diet foods and exercise programs helped? The obesity rate among American adults hit 38 percent in 2015 — a three percent increase from 2012. For the first time in history, researchers note that worldwide, obese people outnumber those who are underweight (The Lancet).

A 2014 study found that 10 percent of Americans consume 25 percent or more of their daily calories in the form of added sugars (JAMA). The average American eats 152 pounds of refined sugar a year. That's 22 teaspoons of sugar everyday (and kids even more).

You'd consume more than that amount in two-12-ounce cans of soda (9.6 teaspoons per can) and 1/4 a doughnut (2.5 teaspoons). Recommendations are to eat no more than 6 teaspoons daily, and less if possible.

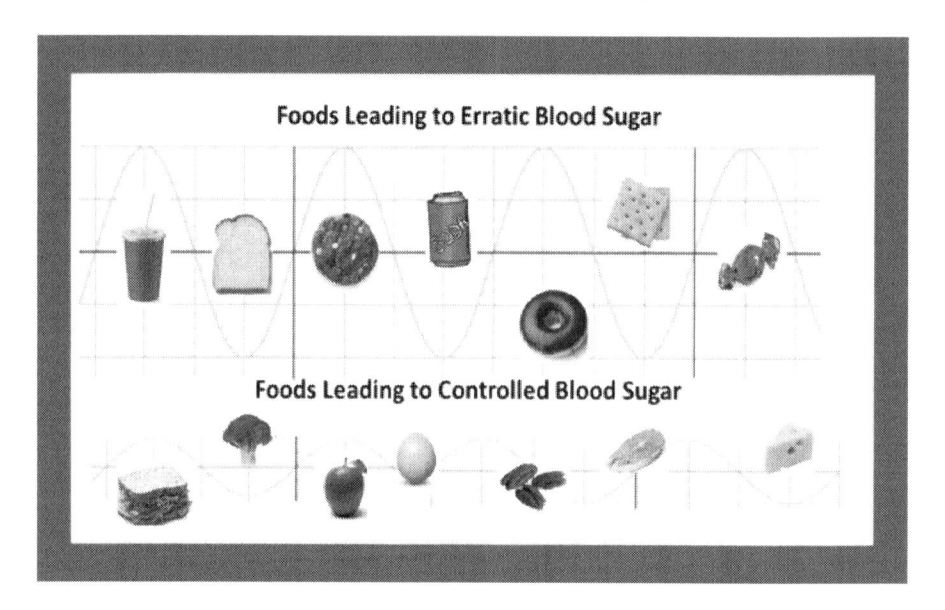

Michele Obamas Let's Move Campaign
Michele Obama's "Let's Move" campaign was a failure, in terms of making a dent in childhood obesity and related diseases. Research shows childhood obesity continued to worsen after the launch of this nationwide program in 2010 with severe obesity rising the most (JAMA).

Essentially, the program didn't focus on the source of the problem – highly sugared, toxic and processed foods – rather focused on exercising more. Make no mistake. The food industry does not want you off sugar or their processed foods.

Dire Consequences for Kids
The ramifications of our high-sugar consumption are dire. "We are now seeing heart attacks in children as young as 8. We're seeing 30-year-olds on kidney dialysis after suffering kidney failure. Type 2 diabetes in American adolescents in 1980 was zero. Indeed, type 2 diabetes was referred to as adult-onset diabetes and was historically unheard of in children and young adults. However, in 2010, nearly 57,640 American adolescents were diagnosed with type 2 diabetes," reports the Mercola.com website.

The fact is that one-third of American kids ages 2 and 19 are now overweight or obese, and that means that chronic disease and mortality rates will skyrocket in coming decades.

Metabolizing Sugary and Carbohydrate-Rich Foods
Let's get some perspective on the sugared foods we eat. One 20-ounce soda would require over an hour of exercise to burn off. You're looking at a 20-minute jog to burn up just one chocolate chip cookie. And a medium order of French Fries? Hit the road for an hour.

When you choose whole foods like nuts, seeds, grains and vegetables, you have a slower rise in blood sugar and less insulin release. This also results in less stored fat in the cells. By the way, hold that soft drink! It contains high fructose corn syrup which is metabolized entirely by your liver. The calories are turned directly into body fat.

1. *How much sugar do you and your family consume?*
   _____
   _____
   _____

2. *Overconsumption of sugar is related to many lifestyle diseases. Discuss with the group steps you could take to slash your consumption.*
   _____
   _____
   _____

Keep in mind that it generally takes three to four days for the blood sugar to stabilize once you make a choice to give up the refined, white foods. Stick with it! The cravings will pass (after a few days, the brownie you thought you just *had* to have becomes more resistible).

Topic #2

LIFESTYLE DISEASES – THE ONE'S WE CAUSE

Not just obesity, but now – more than ever – we are seeing diseases directly related to eating so many refined and processed foods in America. They are called the *diseases of lifestyle*. These are chronic, which means they are ongoing. And they are generally preventable.

Unlike infectious diseases that we *catch,* diseases of lifestyle are brought on by our choices. Arthritis, diabetes, heart disease, cancer, obesity and cancer are examples. They are responsible for seven out of every 10 deaths in the U.S. (CDC).

1. As caring parents, grandparents or concerned individuals, do you think it is time to take responsibility for our health, making choices that will keep us – and our loved ones – out of harm's way?
   _____
   _____

2. Think of examples of infectious diseases you and your family have experienced (chickenpox, flu, colds).
   _____
   _____

3. *Do you or your family have any lifestyle diseases like arthritis, heart disease, diabetes, etc.?*

   _____
   _____
   _____

Topic #3

Digestion – Key to Health

The Digestive Tract

Think of the digestive tract as *a little of the outside running through your insides*. Digestion starts when you smell, see or even *hear* sounds – like meat sizzling on the BBQ or a potato chip bag being opened.

Once you begin chewing, important enzymes are released in the saliva that start digestion. When you don't chew your food well, you lose the advantage of these important enzymes and large chunks of food enter your stomach, partially chewed.

Proper chewing allows you to absorb more nutrition and leads to less gas, belching, bloating and burping. Practice chewing your food until it is liquefied and has lost all its texture – 20 to 30 chomps a bite.

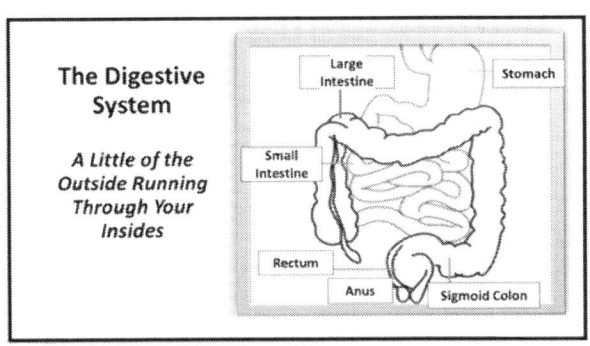

The Digestive System

A Little of the Outside Running Through Your Insides

(Diagram labels: Large Intestine, Stomach, Small Intestine, Rectum, Anus, Sigmoid Colon)

Hydrochloric Acid

When food reaches the stomach, it is mixed with Hydrochloric Acid (HcL) and the enzyme Pepsin. When you don't have these secretions, your food doesn't get broken down well. The result? Belch, bloat and burp, and a loss of important nutrients.

Many people think they have digestive issues because of too much stomach acid. In fact, they may not have enough, so the food begins to ferment in the stomach. A complete digestive enzyme in supplemental form, taken with meals, may help if you have digestive problems.

Be aware of how much longer it takes to chew and swallow whole foods like nuts, seeds and salad, versus a doughnut. Because the whole foods have fiber, they simply require more time before swallowing.

1. *Do you chew your food well? What can you do to chew food until it is liquified? Could you count the chews? Make a game of it at the dinner table and everyone count their chews?*

   _____
   _____
   _____

Topic #4

INFLAMMATION – THE START OF ALL DISEASES

Every chronic disease is associated with inflammation. The American diet is "rich in pro-inflammatory compounds, while lacking antioxidants and other nutrients that help prevent and control inflammation," *(Arizona Center for Advanced Medicine)*. In later videos, we will be talking a lot more about the American diet and how it causes inflammation.

1. *For now, think about what pro-inflammatory foods you eat on a daily basis. These are packaged, processed, sugared, low-nutrition, preserved foods.*

   _____
   _____
   _____

2. *Share with your group what steps you can take to lower your intake of these pro-inflammatory foods.*

   _____
   _____
   _____

Healthy Foods Mentioned in the Bible

Apples, Almonds, Dates, Figs, Grapes, Melons, Olives, Pistachio Nuts, Pomegranates, Raisins, Sycamore Fruit, Beans, Cucumbers, Gourds, Leeks, Lentils, Onions, Barley, Bread, Millet, Spelt, Unleavened Bread, Wheat, Fish, Partridge, Pigeon, Quail, Dove, Calf, Goat, Lamb, Sheep, Venison, Butter, Cheese, Curds, Milk, Eggs, Grape Juice, Honey, Locust, Olive Oil, Vinegar, Wine, Anise, Coriander, Cinnamon, Cumin, Dill, Garlic, Mint, Mustard, Rue, Salt.

1. *Do you see any processed foods on the list?*
   _____
   _____
   _____

I Wish Above All Things That You May Prosper and be in Health, Even as Thy Soul Prospers
3 John 2:1

Video #2

Topic #1

The Bones

Just like your muscles and organs, the bones are living tissue and require exercise and nutrients to stay strong and healthy. The very best type of exercise to strengthen bones is anything that is weight-bearing.

This includes lifting weights, walking, hiking, jogging, climbing stairs, tennis, and dancing. These kinds of movement work the tendons that attach muscle to bone, which in turn, boosts bone strength. While swimming and bicycling are great sports, they aren't weight-bearing because they don't work against gravity.

1. *What weight-bearing exercises do you do? How could you incorporate them into your daily routine if you are not already doing them?*

_____
_____
_____

Osteoporosis

Like all the diseases of lifestyle, osteoporosis – a condition where the bones become porous and riddled with holes – is on the rise. According to the *National*

Osteoporosis Foundation, over 50 million Americans have this disease, or low bone density.

It is called "the silent disease" because bone loss usually occurs gradually over the years, without symptoms. People with osteoporosis can break a bone from a minor fall or even from a simple action like sneezing or bumping into furniture.

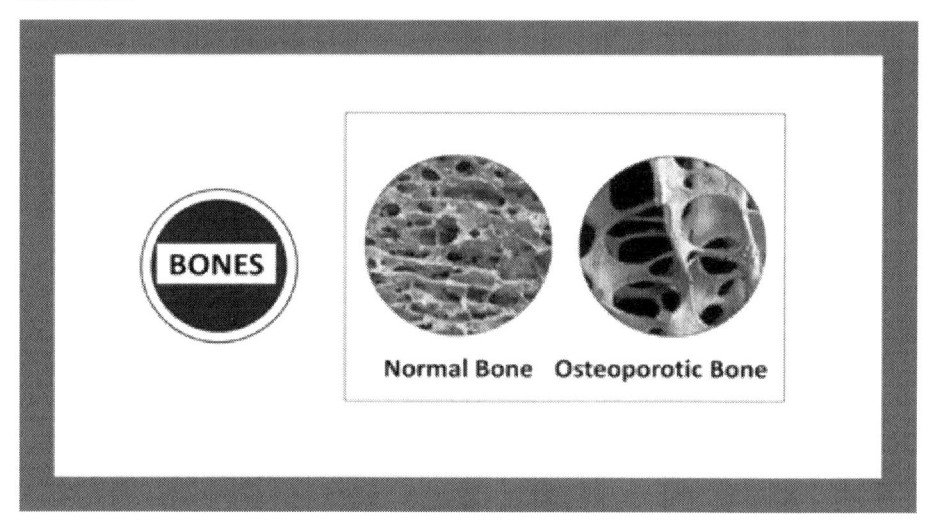

1. *Can you see from the picture how weak and vulnerable your bones can become if they don't get the nutrients they need?*

   _____
   _____
   _____

Keeping Bones Strong

In addition to weight-bearing exercises, you should be eating whole foods that are bone-friendly and nutrient dense. These are the foods that don't come in shiny, metallic packages with glitzy labels. Rather, they are whole, natural foods of color like salmon, blueberries, spinach, apples, beets, etc.

It's common knowledge that the bones need calcium. For people who don't like or are allergic to milk, it's good to know you can get calcium in other foods. For example, kale, sardines, broccoli, watercress, bok choy, okra and almonds are great sources.

More Bone Friendly Nutrients

Vitamin D – found in hazelnuts, figs, sardines, eggs, dark and leafy greens, broccoli and wild caught salmon – is needed for calcium absorption. And vitamin K – present in dark, leafy greens and peas – is critical for the entire bone matrix.

A lesser known mineral – manganese – is involved in making strong bone mass. It's found in pineapple, almonds, pecans and oatmeal. Pineapples are a particularly good source of manganese.

1. *Of the foods mentioned above, how many of them do you eat on a regular basis? Consider that two liters of soft drinks cost about the same as a fresh pineapple. Why do you think fresh pineapple and a glass of pure water is a better choice over soft drinks?*

   _____
   _____
   _____

Topic #2

TEXT NECK - 21ST CENTURY AILMENT

There is an alarming new condition – *Text Neck* – that is being seen frequently. According to recent research, text neck results from the poor posture people assume when texting. Over time, this posture can lead to early wear-and-tear on the spine, degeneration and even surgery.

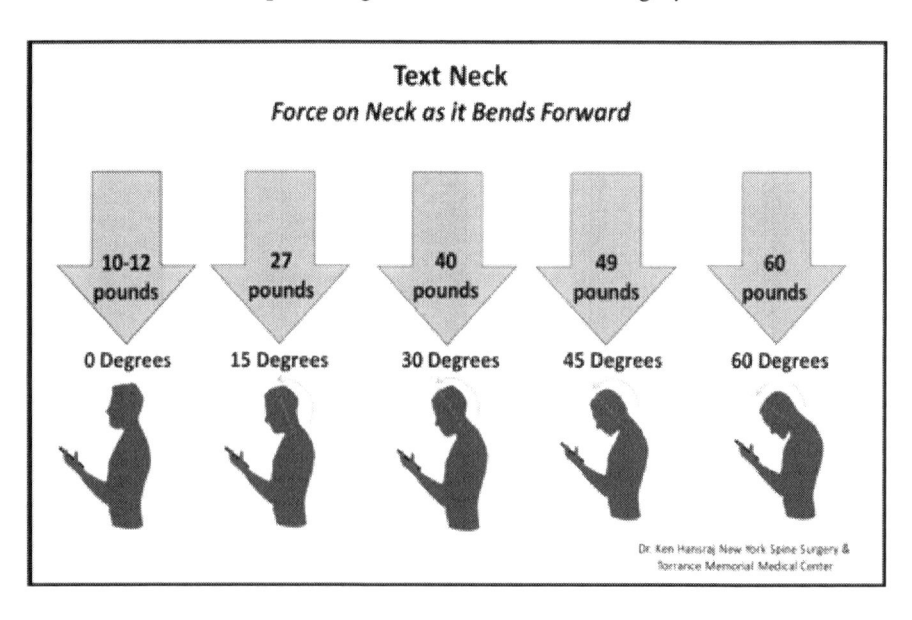

Text Neck
Force on Neck as it Bends Forward

10-12 pounds	27 pounds	40 pounds	49 pounds	60 pounds
0 Degrees	15 Degrees	30 Degrees	45 Degrees	60 Degrees

Dr. Ken Hansraj New York Spine Surgery & Torrance Memorial Medical Center

How to Survive the American High-Tech Diet

"It is an epidemic," according to Ken Hansraj, chief surgeon at *New York Spine Surgery*. As the neck bends forward and down, up to 60 pounds of extra weight can be placed on the spine. It would be like carrying around a 60-pound child on your neck for several hours a day." Get your head up! Hold the phone at a 70-90° angle to the body.

1. *Observe how people hold their cell phone and the downward slant of their neck and back. Do you see your children in this position?*
   _____
   _____

2. *How do you think you would feel after carrying a 60-pound child on your neck for a few hours?*
   _____
   _____

Topic #3

Human Organs

The Kidneys

The *kidneys* require plenty of pure water. Unfortunately, many people live on mostly soft drinks and caffeinated beverages, shunning wholesome water. A good rule of thumb: divide your body weight in half and drink that many ounces of water a day. Lemons are a natural kidney detoxifier. Ask for lemons to go with your water when eating out.

For *bladder infections* – in addition to commonly known remedies like cranberries – there is a natural substance called D-Mannose that is beneficial. In 2014, researchers reported in the *World Journal of Urology* that D-mannose powder could significantly decrease the risk of recurrent urinary tract infections. It's E. coli that causes 90% of urinary tract infections. D-Mannose – when taken as a supplement - attaches to the bacteria, allowing it to become easily expelled.

The Adrenal Glands

Think of your *adrenals* as the energy glands. Often, people with weak adrenal glands get dizzy when they squat down, then stand up suddenly. There is an easy way to test your adrenals.

James Balch MD writes, "Take and compare two blood pressure readings – one lying down and one while standing. First lie down and rest for five minutes. Then take your blood pressure. Stand up and immediately take your blood pressure again. If your blood pressure reading is lower after standing up, suspect reduced adrenal gland function."

Vitamin C and B5 (*pantothenic acid*) are very supportive to the adrenals. I personally suffered with weak adrenals years back and got better by aggressively following an organic vegetable juicing program. I focused on vegetables rich in pantothenic acid and vitamin C: endive, cucumbers, lemons and dark leafy greens.

1. *Here are some pantothenic-acid-rich foods: brewer's yeast, black strap molasses, eggs, legumes, mushrooms, nuts, royal jelly (made by honey bees), avocado, filbert nuts, broccoli and whole wheat. Do you frequently eat these foods?*

_____
_____
_____

The Gallbladder

Gallstones can be caused by food sensitivity, and the top three foods that cause symptoms are eggs, pork, and onions, according to researcher Alan R. Gaby. MD. Removing these foods from the diet for just one week can bring relief from gallbladder pain—and prevent unnecessary surgery, he says.

In my clinical experience, I have found that many other foods are suspect. Consider having food sensitivity testing done, or follow the "at-home" testing described in video #4. A sample of how to record test results *is available on the website at "products and services on videos" tab.*

The Liver

Each year, more than 4 billion pounds of chemical compounds are released into the environment, added to food or poured into water. Produce is sprayed with toxic chemicals, and animals are injected with hormones and antibiotics. The liver must cope with these toxic chemicals as it is the main blood filter in the body.

Add to that the poor diets we eat, the liver simply becomes overburdened. It's a good idea to occasionally undertake a detoxification program. A good metabolic detoxification program will provide liver-specific nutrients to encourage the elimination of unwanted chemicals from your body. And be sure to eat beets, leafy greens, garlic, lemons, turmeric and green tea.

The Heart

The heart can benefit from magnesium-rich foods – spinach, chard, pumpkin seeds, yogurt, almonds and black beans. Further, the grain *buckwheat* contains a bioflavonoid called *Rutin*. Rutin – well known for its ties to a healthy heart and vascular system – it's abundant in buckwheat (soba noodles, cereals).

Nobel-prize work was done in 1998 that identified *Nitric Oxide* as a critical component for heart health. Without Nitric Oxide, there is no life. Nitric oxide is a signaling molecule that helps blood vessels relax and open to increase circulation. The amino acid L-arginine causes the body to make more of it. Foods sources of L-arginine are seafood, soy and spinach.

1. *Do you ever eat buckwheat? Try using it to make pancakes. Buckwheat "ramen" type noodles are available in natural food stores.*
   _____
   _____
   _____

1. *In a 10-year study on 30,000 Seventh Day Adventists, it was found that those who consumed raw nuts at least five times weekly had a 48% lower risk of death from Coronary Heart Disease. Do you eat whole, raw unsalted nuts?*
   _____
   _____
   _____

How to Survive the American High-Tech Diet

1. *Foods with flavonoids and foods with color are heart healthy. These include deeply colored fruits and vegetables. Is your diet rich in these foods?*

   _____
   _____
   _____

Topic #4

Exercising Against Gravity

Dr. Joan Vernikos – exercise physiologist to the astronauts – began working with NASA during the *Skylab* program. She noted that astronauts aged prematurely while in space, much the way a person ages when bedridden.

In fact, changes in bone and muscle that occur here on Earth in one year's time occur in just one week to one month when you're in space. She explains that there is a 10-fold acceleration of aging because of the gravity-free environment!

"What became abundantly clear to me very quickly was that gravity plays a big role in our physiological function and in the aging process," writes Dr. Vernikos. She recommends standing up over 30 times a day as a powerful antidote to long periods of sitting. There are unlimited opportunities for movement all day long – housework, gardening, even cooking. Her book, *"Sitting Kills Moving Heals,"* is a worthy read!

1. *What "against-gravity" exercises do you do. Get up and move frequently – several times an hour, even if it's just for a minute.*

   _____
   _____
   _____

One Key to Eating Healthy: Avoid Anything That Has a TV Commercial

Video #3

Topic #1

Healthy Eyes

Think "*fresh, wild and colorful*" when choosing foods to nourish your eyes. Foods of vibrant color are chockful of potent natural substances called carotenoids. *Lutein* and *Zeaxanthin* are two carotenoids that have been proven to nourish and strengthen the eyes, and keep vision sharp.

Foods rich in Lutein and Zeaxanthin include blueberries, kale, paprika, spinach, collards, mustard greens, turnip greens and Swiss chard. Give some of the more "unusual" dark leafy greens a try in salads or cooked in soups and stews. They can be tough, but you can tenderize them for salads by removing the stem, then massaging the leaves a few moments to break down the fibers (save the stems for juicing).

1. *Why would a meal of grilled Alaskan salmon, Caesar salad with romaine lettuce and fresh blueberries be healthier for the eyes than hot dogs, cola and doughnuts?*
   _____
   _____
   _____

2. *Do you ever eat eye-health-promoting Swiss chard, mustard greens, turnip greens or collard greens? Discuss with the group ideas of how to cook them.*
   _____
   _____
   _____

3. *Are you beginning to see the importance of eating whole foods?*
   _____
   _____
   _____

Topic #2

HEALTHY SKIN

For healthy skin, you'll want to watch out for AGE's, or *advanced glycation end products*. But never mind the scientific name, these are inflammation-causing, age-promoting molecules that form when sugar meets protein and fat. The combination creates the perfect storm!

High Fructose Corn Syrup is an extremely potent pro-inflammatory agent that creates AGEs and speeds up the aging process. Researchers in *Israel* have shown that excessive consumption of fructose accelerates the production of AGEs and causes your skin to be less resistant to wrinkles. Soft drinks are major culprit. Get off them – and sugar in general.

Topic #3

THE BRAIN

Not to sound like a broken record, but sugar rears its ugly head again! Researchers now call Alzheimer's Disease *Diabetes #3*. They say it is caused by a lifetime of eating too many refined carbohydrates, too much sugar and not enough "healthy" fat. A lifelong diet of eating these sugary foods starts the "brain-damage cascade" long before the disease ever manifests.

Sugar promotes inflammation. "If you looked at an autopsy of a brain of an Alzheimer's patient, you'd see a brain on fire. This inflammation occurs over-and-over again in every chronic disease and very dramatically with the aging brain and overall aging process," researcher Mark Hyman MD writes.

The good news is you can reverse the process. Cut sugars and refined carbs to control your insulin and balance your blood sugar levels - *NOW!* Don't wait until the disease begins to manifest

1. *There it is again! That age-old enemy – sugar. Find ways to greatly reduce it in your diet. Discuss ideas with your group.*
   _____
   _____
   _____

Topic #4

WAISTWATCHERSWINNERS.COM

Change the Way You Think

The main topic of video #3 is weight loss. It's Dr. Phil who said, "Successful weight loss requires programming, not willpower." What an accurate statement! Forty-five million Americans go on a diet each year and spend $33 billion annually on weight loss products. Yet, nearly two-thirds of Americans are overweight or obese. Clearly, diets don't work!

1. *Have you tried to lose weight based strictly on willpower?*
   _____
   _____
   _____

2. *Did hunger win out eventually and you gave in?*
   _____
   _____
   _____

Developing New Habits

Have you seen Marie on TV advertising a major weight loss program? They provide you with all your favorites – lasagna, pizza and brownies – but they don't teach you how to change your habits. You can stick with these types of programs and possibly lose some weight, but in the end, you'll most likely go back to old eating habits because the program has not taught you how to make changes. Why? Losing the weight is only part of the problem. Deciding "to" and learning "how" to change old habits is far more likely to lead to lifelong success.

1. *What would happen if you went on a nationally advertised weight loss program, lost the weight, then went back to your regular diet?*
   _____
   _____
   _____

2. *Have you done that before?*
   _____
   _____
   _____

Change Your Brain

I recently developed a program called *Waist Watchers Winners* to help people change the way they think about food. It is 60 days of motivation delivered via email daily. The lessons can apply to weight loss, but are also very effective for helping you change any undesired habit.

Why 60 days? Doctors and neuroscientists know that it takes that long to really change a habit. What's that you say? Sixty days you ask? Yes, it seems like a long time, but when you compare it to the years you may have been carrying extra weight or repeating an unwanted habit, it's not long at all. The bottom line is: successful, lifelong weight loss requires changing habits, ideas and thinking – not just starving.

The WaistWatchersWinners.com lessons are short and can be completed in just a few minutes. They are designed to help you change how you think about food. If you are interested, you can get the first three days for free at the website (HealthTreasureChest.com).

1. *Think about all the different diets you've tried in your life. As for me, I can think of well over a dozen different programs. If so inclined, discuss different diets that you have tried.*

   _____
   _____
   _____

Process of Change

This ladder of achievement really shows the process of change. If you'll begin to change the way you "think" you can make permanent changes in unwanted habits. The first step: be willing to ask, "*what is it.*" As I've experienced clinically, when a person says *I won't,* they aren't interested in doing anything differently.

Ladder of Achievement

I did
I can
I think I can
I might
I think I might
What is it?
I don't know how
I can't
I won't

1. *Where are you on this ladder?*

   _____
   _____

2. Do you have weight you'd like to lose or a habit you'd like to change?
   _____
   _____

3. Make a goal for the change you would like to make.
   _____
   _____

4. Make your goal SMART ("I'm going to lose 50 pounds in the two weeks before my high school reunion" is none of these!). SMART stands for:
   a. Specific (I will follow a low-fat diet and increase my exercise)
   b. Measurable (I will weigh once a week and write down the weight)
   c. Achievable (I can achieve this because I will plan ahead for meals)
   d. Realistic (20 pounds in four months is realistic)
   e. Timely (This is good timing because the kids will be back in school)

Years ago, I jogged on a private runway. I don't really like jogging, so I used goalsetting to get through the drudgery. I'd focus on the telephone pole just ahead. When I reached it, I'd look to the next pole. It really helped me set "short term" goals to reach my "long term" target.

Triangles and Habits

The three triangles viewed on the video #3 demonstrate how we develop habits and then repeat them without thinking. You might have habits like: eating a doughnut at work because it's what you've always done; cleaning your plate because that's what you were taught as a child; always overeating at a buffet because the food is free. Changing habits generally requires a new way of looking at things.

Habits

Much like brushing teeth, we develop habits and repeat them without thinking – over and over and day after day. These phrases are an example. Most people read them incorrectly – the way they've come to "learn" to read them.

- A Bird in the the Hand
- Spring Time in in Paris
- Once in a a Life Time

Learning New Habits Requires Deciding to Look at Things a New Way

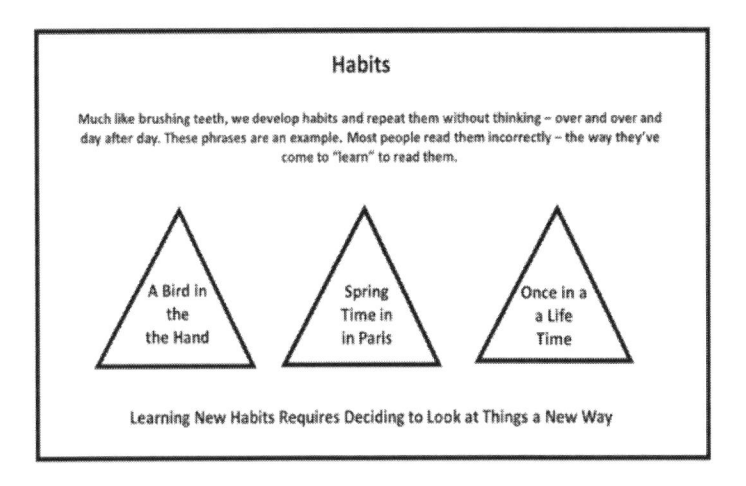

Eating Triggers

For most of us, the well-known phrase "see food eat food" applies. It's automatic eating, or repeating what we've always done. The problem is, automatic eating can lead to overeating, which leads to overweight.

An automatic eater eats from habit. They never give a thought to the consequences of indulging. A sophisticated eater tends to think about food before they eat. They might ask themselves, "Do I need it? Am I really hungry? Will there be consequences? Could I eat something else to keep from indulging in that fattening cake?"

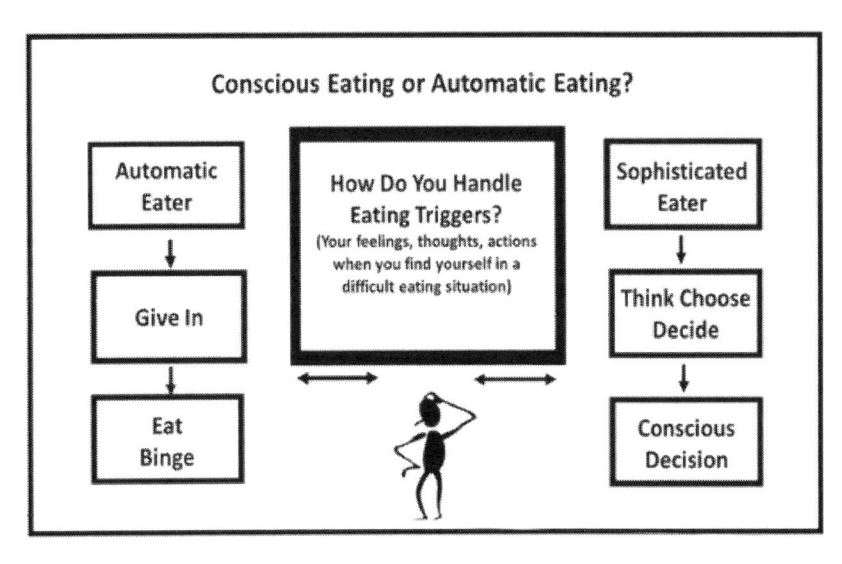

Conscious Eating or Automatic Eating?

Automatic Eater → Give In → Eat Binge

How Do You Handle Eating Triggers?
(Your feelings, thoughts, actions when you find yourself in a difficult eating situation)

Sophisticated Eater → Think Choose Decide → Conscious Decision

1. Which are you? An automatic eater or a sophisticated eater?
   _____
   _____

2. Do you ever stop and think about what you are about to put in your mouth and the consequences?
   _____
   _____
   _____

The Domino Effect

Automatic eaters give in when they've eaten something they shouldn't, when they "slip." Then they might gorge, thinking they will restart their diet tomorrow. They repeat this habit week after week, year after year.

A sophisticated eater is more likely to recover after a slip. If they eat something they wished they hadn't, they get right back on track.

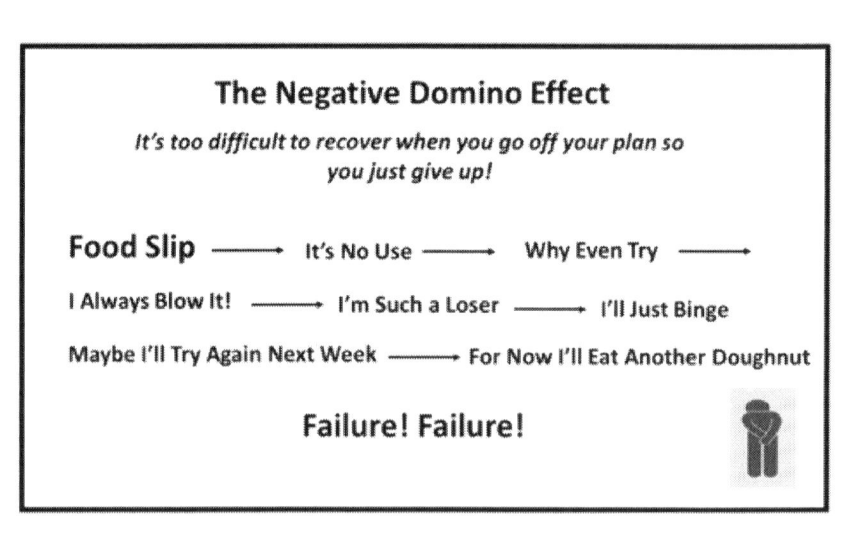

The Negative Domino Effect

It's too difficult to recover when you go off your plan so you just give up!

Food Slip ⟶ It's No Use ⟶ Why Even Try ⟶

I Always Blow It! ⟶ I'm Such a Loser ⟶ I'll Just Binge

Maybe I'll Try Again Next Week ⟶ For Now I'll Eat Another Doughnut

Failure! Failure!

> **The Positive Domino Effect**
>
> *You realize you will have "slips." When it happens, you get right back on track.*
>
> **Food Slip!**
>
> I Didn't Mean to Eat That ⟶ I'm Still on Track ⟶ It's OK
>
> I'm Doing Great! ⟶ I'm Down 20 Pounds ⟶
>
> **Success! Success!**

These are just a few examples of the 60 lessons available at **WaistWatchersWinners.com**. I hope you'll join me on the adventure and have great success!

A Five Chapter Story
Chapter 1
I was walking down the street. There was a big hole. I fell in. It wasn't my fault. It took me a long time to get out.
Chapter 2
I was walking down the street. There was a big hole. I fell in. It wasn't my fault. I got out quickly.
Chapter 3
I was walking down the street. There was a big hole. I fell in. It *was* my fault. I got out quickly.
Chapter 4
I was walking down the street. There was a big hole. I walked around it.
Chapter 5
I took another street.

Video #4

Topic #1

THINKING OUTSIDE THE BOX

We ended video #3 with the nine-dot puzzle. It's an example of *thinking outside the box*. This puzzle was originally designed to help people learn to "think" differently. The point is that we get trapped in old ways of thinking, which is problematic if the thoughts are counterproductive.

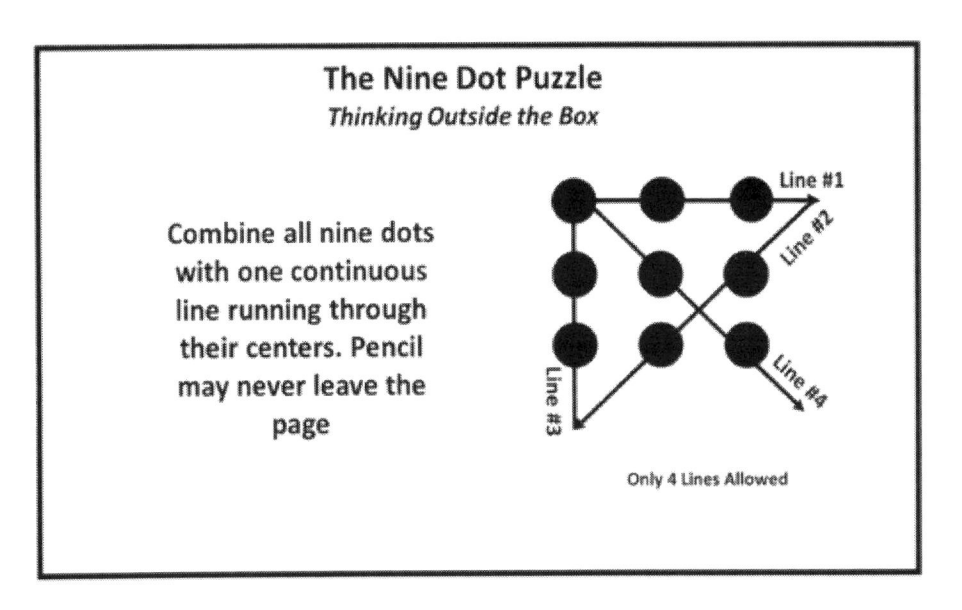

The Nine Dot Puzzle
Thinking Outside the Box

Combine all nine dots with one continuous line running through their centers. Pencil may never leave the page

Only 4 Lines Allowed

Many of our habits lead us down a destructive road – one that is filled with potholes and traps. Sometimes to solve a problem, you need to remove assumptions you've made and be willing to look at things in a new way.

1. *Did you solve the nine-dot puzzle? Did it represent any other meanings to you?*
   _____
   _____
   _____

Applying the Nine-Dot Puzzle to Weight Loss

When it comes to losing weight, the nine-dot puzzle is an analogy. To lose weight "for life," you must be willing to try new things, to adjust your ideas about dieting and food and eating. It will probably involve "unlearning" some of your troublesome habits.

1. *Can you think of any "locked-in" thoughts you have about food or eating? (An example: I must load up my plate at a buffet because the food is free).*
   _____
   _____

2. *If weight is not an issue for you, can you think of any locked-in ideas you could benefit from changing?*
   _____
   _____

3. *Below are a few examples of faulty thinking. How could you change and improve the thinking? I'll complete the first two (if you don't have a weight problem, apply the principles to a habit you'd like to change):*
   _____
   _____
   _____

- *I have always eaten quickly and can't help it – If I eat more slowly, I will be able to savor each bite.*
- *My eating pattern in ingrained and unchangeable – I have control over my behaviors and can learn a new eating style with some effort and practice.*
- *I can't help what I do; it's the way I was raised –*
- *I should eat this now before someone else gets it –*
- *I should never throw food away –*
- *I won't enjoy eating as much if I eat differently –*
- *No matter what I do I put on weight –*
- *I should eat this before it becomes stale –*
- *I only like certain kinds of foods –*

Changing Up Your Day

Are you ready to try something new? Pick the one habit you'd like to change, then decide on another behavior you could do instead. Here is the example used in the video: rather than getting up, brewing coffee and going to your computer, try making a glass of fresh vegetable juice and doing 10 squats. Then, go for your coffee and computer.

1. *What could you do differently that would be beneficial? It doesn't need to be a major change – just something that will begin to break your "learned" routine.*

   _____
   _____
   _____

2. *Once you decide, do you think you can make yourself do it daily until it becomes automatic?*

   _____
   _____
   _____

Topic #2

What Have They Done to Our Food?

Really, it's criminal what's been done to our food. If a turn of the century American was suddenly propelled into a modern supermarket, they'd be aghast at the thousands of different products that grace the shelves. Here are just a few examples of what's done to our food:

- In the past five decades, **Food Additive** usage has skyrocketed from about 800 to more than 10,000 substances. They are added to everything from baked goods and breakfast cereals to energy bars and carbonated drinks. *(npr.org.)*
- Fifteen million pounds of **Artificial Food Dyes** are poured into the U.S. food supply annually; some are linked to cancer and hyperactivity in children. *(CSPI).*
- **Emulsifiers** make foods like ice cream and salad dressings creamy. When immunologist Andrew Gewirtz and his colleagues fed common emulsifiers to mice, they became obese and developed glucose intolerance. (*Nature Journal Science* 2015).
- **Artificial Sweeteners** are associated with numerous health problems. Look at the illustration.

How to Survive the American High-Tech Diet

A Few of 91 Symptoms Reported to FDA from Aspartame Consumption

Anxiety	Arthritis	Heart Palpitations
Candida	Asthma	Hair Loss
Obesity	Bloating	Hives
Headache	Edema	HPB
Tooth Decay	Seizures	Impotency
ADHD	Chronic Fatigue	Insomnia
Diabetes	Chronic Cough	Itching
Mood Swings	Confusion	Joint Pain
Brain Lesions	Candida	Brain Fog
Brain Tumors	Diarrhea	Memory Loss
Depression	Dizziness	Muscle Spasms
Swelling	Flushing	Weight Gain

The bottom line is: when you eat processed and packaged foods, you are consuming a plethora of artificial ingredients. Many have been scientifically proven to cause disease.

1. *Can you see the advantage of staying away from processed foods?*
   _____
   _____

2. *What choices can you make in cutting down on processed foods?*
   _____
   _____
   _____

Boxed and Packaged Foods

Look at the label from a popular variety of boxed au gratin potatoes. It contains 29 different ingredients. A baked potato contains one ingredient: potato.

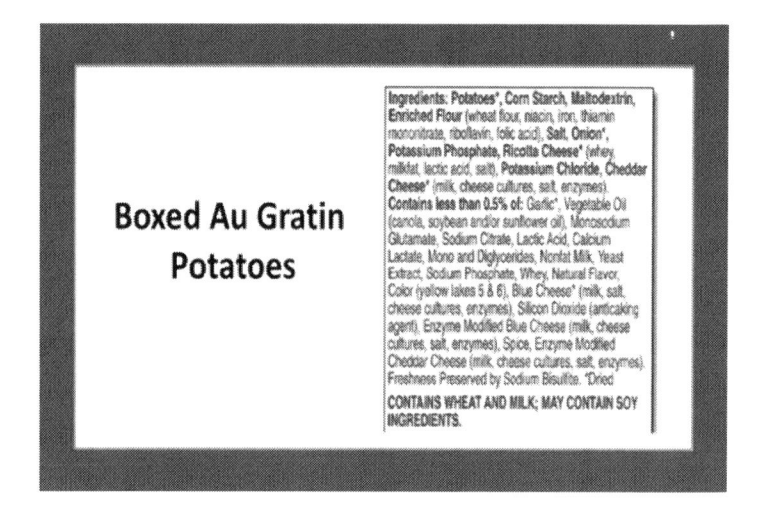

Boxed Au Gratin Potatoes

Ingredients: Potatoes*, Corn Starch, Maltodextrin, Enriched Flour (wheat flour, niacin, iron, thiamin mononitrate, riboflavin, folic acid), **Salt, Onion*, Potassium Phosphate, Ricotta Cheese*** (whey, milkfat, lactic acid, salt), **Potassium Chloride, Cheddar Cheese*** (milk, cheese cultures, salt, enzymes). **Contains less than 0.5% of:** Garlic*, Vegetable Oil (canola, soybean and/or sunflower oil), Monosodium Glutamate, Sodium Citrate, Lactic Acid, Calcium Lactate, Mono and Diglycerides, Nonfat Milk, Yeast Extract, Sodium Phosphate, Whey, Natural Flavor, Color (yellow lakes 5 & 6), Blue Cheese* (milk, salt, cheese cultures, enzymes), Silicon Dioxide (anticaking agent), Enzyme Modified Blue Cheese (milk, cheese cultures, salt, enzymes), Spice, Enzyme Modified Cheddar Cheese (milk cheese cultures, salt, enzymes). Freshness Preserved by Sodium Bisulfite. *Dried **CONTAINS WHEAT AND MILK; MAY CONTAIN SOY INGREDIENTS.**

1. *How many different ingredients do you think you might be eating in a meal of frozen chicken nuggets, boxed au gratin potatoes and a fried apple pie?*

   _____
   _____
   _____

2. *What about an organic chicken breast, a baked potato and an apple?*

   _____
   _____
   _____

Popular Kids Cereals

The next time you shop, notice where the highly advertised kid's cereals are located. In a study of 65 cereals in 10 different grocery stores, Cornell researchers found that cereals marketed to kids are placed half as high on shelves as adult cereals. (foodpsychology.cornell.edu).

The Problem with Fiber-less Foods

Not only are our foods artificial, they are devoid of fiber. Denis Burkitt, MD (1911-1993) spent many years in Africa studying the diets of rural Africans.

His research showed that native Africans who eat whole, natural, high fiber foods have three times the elimination as his average English counterpart.

He also noted they do not get the lifestyle diseases of modern civilization: heart disease, cancer, arthritis, hemorrhoids etc. He concluded that their diet – high in fiber and nutrient-rich – not only provided more nutrition, but raced through their digestive system rapidly. They were simply less toxic. His book is, *Don't Forget Fiber in Your Diet.*

1. *Is your diet rich in fiber?*

   _____

   _____

2. *How is your elimination system? Some of Dr. Burkitt's English friends only eliminated once a week. Africans eliminate after nearly every meal because of their high fiber diet.*

   _____

   _____

3. *What do you think rural Africans eat? Would it be artificially colored or flavored? Boxed? Microwavable? Fiberless?*

   _____

   _____

   _____

Topic #3

ONE INGREDIENT FOODS

For good health and weight loss, stick with "one ingredient foods" or combinations of them, most of the time. By doing this, you will avoid the additives found in processed and packaged foods. You'll find these foods along the periphery of the grocery aisles. Avoid the center aisles where all the packaged and processed foods are located.

1. *Do you eat many one-ingredient foods or combinations of them?*
   _____
   _____
   _____

2. *Check out your cupboards this week and read the labels on some of the packaged foods.*
   _____
   _____
   _____

Lisa's Story

Lisa was 100 pounds overweight, depressed and tired. She was a nurse and her legs and feet were killing her – all the time. She desperately wanted to get well. So, to the Tahoma Clinic she came.

When she made her way into my office, I could see that she wasn't doing well. As always, I started by asking her what she ate. She said she was addicted to diet soda. "I drink it all day long. Maybe 7-8 cans." Top that with mostly boxed food, her diet was leading her down a path of health "destruction." She had no idea that Aspartame is thought by many naturally-oriented health professionals to be the most dangerous additive in our food.

Lisa was compliant to my suggestions. Almost immediately, she began to lose weight. Lots of weight! She reached her goal and is in great health today.

Topic #4

FOOD SENSITIVITIES

The final topic on this video is food sensitivities. I saw so many people at the Tahoma Clinic who were reacting to the food they ate. But somehow, they'd never made any association between their diet and nagging symptoms such as headache, stomachache, mental confusion, fatigue and sleepiness (and there are many more). And the foods that were the worse culprits? Eggs, milk, wheat and soy.

There are plenty of books available to help you sort through food allergies at home. If you'd like to do a blood test that provides accurate results based on your blood, consider the ALCAT Blood Test (antigen leukocyte antibody test). You can read about it on the website (www.healthtreasurechest.com).

The ALCAT will introduce your blood to up to 450 different foods and substances. When your body does not like a food, the white blood cells expand and leak, leading to nagging symptoms. Once your sensitivities are determined, you are given an individualized diet based on your results and a private phone consultation.

Testing at Home for Food Sensitivities

Below is a sample chart of how you can track your food sensitivities (there is a larger sample on the website). Here is how it works. Each meal is only ONE food.

How to Survive the American High-Tech Diet

No condiments. Salt OK. Eat until comfortably full. Eat each food alone – with nothing else – so you can pinpoint symptoms (for example, if you eat a casserole with 15 ingredients, you won't know which food you are reacting to).

Sit calmly for a few minutes, then take your pulse. Eat the food. Then, take your pulse at wrist or neck at 15, 30, 45 minutes and 1 hour. Watch for symptoms: headache, stomachache, confusion, itching, mood swing etc. If your pulse goes up or down by 10 points after eating a food – or if you have negative symptoms – remove that food from your diet for 3-6 months. Once you have identified a food as "safe," you can begin adding it – in combination – with other "safe" foods.

MONDAY FOOD	Pulse Before Eating	Pulse 15 min	Pulse 30 min	Pulse 45 min	Pulse 1 Hour	Record Any Symptoms: headache, stomach ache, achy, confusion, mood swings, itching, irritable, etc.
Oatmeal 8AM	70	88 Achy muscles	88 Still Achy	82 Pain Better	88 Headache	Didn't feel good for hours after. Still have muscle aches.
Orange 11:30AM	74	80 Good	80 Good	82 Good	80 Good	Oranges seem ok.
Turkey Breast Noon	80	90 Yuck	92 Awful	98 Stomach ache	92 Better	No turkey for me!
Raspberries 3PM	70	80 Good	78 Good	80 Good	82 Good	Felt great with raspberries.
Boiled Eggs 5:30PM	72	88 Itching	88 Achy	90 Achy	90 Went to bed	Eggs made me feel awful. Headache, stomach ache, tired.
Lamb Chop 7PM	80	74 Nothing Unusual	72 Good	72 Good	74 Good	Lamb seems like a good food for me.
Soy Yogurt 9:30PM	78	80 Joints hurt	82 Tired	88 Sleepy	90 Went to bed	No more soy yogurt!

1. *Do you ever feel that you react to foods in a negative way?*
   _____
   _____

2. *What symptoms have you associated with eating specific foods?*
   _____
   _____

3. *What about your children? According to Jonathan Wright MD, "Nearly all children diagnosed with "hyperactivity" have allergies and sensitivities." (More on this in video #8).*

_____
_____
_____

⎯⎯૭⎯⎯

You Can't Change What You Don't Acknowledge
Dr. Phil

Video #5

Topic #1

Juicing for Life

Juicing has become wildly popular in recent years and rightfully so. Freshly squeezed organic juices are a powerhouse of nutrients. I like to think of them as a "liquid vitamin and mineral pill" that is body-ready for quick absorption.

Many of the natural cancer clinics in the world have vegetable juices as part of their protocol. In fact, in one such clinic, the patient's drink a fresh vegetable juice hourly. Notice I say "vegetable" juice. Stay away from fruit juices because of their high sugar content.

Choosing a Juicer

Virtually every authority recommends eating 6-8 vegetables and fruits a day, but not many people reach that recommendation. For anyone interested, I have a juicing E Book on my website: *Juice to Lose*. It has thorough information on juicing, 20 juicing recipes and a meal plan.

When choosing a juicer, make sure is has a pulp extraction tube. With some of the cheaper varieties, the pulp builds up in the juicer and stops the juicing process. You'll find a variety of juicers in department stores or online. We offer a professional juicer – ***the Samson*** – on the website.

1. *Do you have a juicer? Do you use it?*
_____
_____
_____

Topic #2

SENSATIONAL SMOOTHIES

Smoothies can be an excellent meal replacement. And if you don't particularly love dark leafy greens, you can add them to your smoothies. When blended, you won't even notice them! Smoothies are also an excellent way to get powdered and liquid supplements into the diet. Simply add them to the smoothie! Check out the HealthTreasureChest.com Super Smoothie on the website.

Topic #3

Wheatgrass

Considered by many as nature's healthiest beverage, wheatgrass is a powerful, chlorophyll-rich drink. According to the *Optimum Health Institute* in San Diego – a health SPA that provides wheatgrass as part of their daily regimen, "Two ounces of wheatgrass juice has the nutritional equivalent of five pounds of the best raw organic vegetables…twice the amount of Vitamin A as carrots and is higher in Vitamin C than oranges."

"It contains the full spectrum of B vitamins, as well as mega-doses of minerals. Wheatgrass floods the body with therapeutic dosages of antioxidants, enzymes and phytonutrients, and is a powerful detoxifier."

1. *You can make wheatgrass but it requires a specific grinding type of juicer. Many juice bars serve shots of wheatgrass. Do you have a juice bar near you? Give wheatgrass a try.*

    _____
    _____
    _____

Topic #4

Sprouting for Mega-Health

As far back as the 1970s, UCLA studied alfalfa, clover and broccoli sprouts and found that they are 10 times more nutritious than the fully matured vegetable – and some studies say much higher. They are an excellent addition to salads and sandwiches.

Sprouts of all sorts are easy to make at home. There are several sprouting trays and containers on the internet that are easy to use. Keep in mind that sprouts can get moldy, so you'll want to take care when making them.

Rodale's Organic Life website suggests the following cleaning procedure: "One spray bottleful *each* of undiluted white vinegar and undiluted 3% hydrogen peroxide (common drug store variety). Spray seeds first with the vinegar, then with the hydrogen peroxide. Rinse thoroughly." Do this before sprouting.

Topic #5

CELL PHONES

While studies are not conclusive, the health industry is considering the dangers of cell phone radiation. So is the U.S. government. While the studies are coming in, there are several things you can do to limit radiation exposure. According to Dr. Oz (oprah.com):

- *Use a Headset or Speakerphone:* Headsets with cords help reduce risks. These emit much less RF energy, and allow you to move the phone away from your body. One study shows that using a headset lowers radiation exposure eightfold.
- *Keep Your Phone Out of Your Pocket:* A study in the *Journal of Craniofacial Surgery* linked cell phone radiation to decreased bone density in the pelvis, and a 2008 study conducted by the Cleveland Clinic found that it lowers fertility in men.
- *Limit Children's Use:* Kids have a thinner skull, and their brains are still developing.
- *Stop Talking While Driving:* Your cell signal jumps between wireless towers when driving. Since RF is highest when a connection with a tower is first established, talking while traveling can increase exposure.

How to Survive the American High-Tech Diet

- *Don't Chat with a Poor Signal*: The harder your phone must work to get reception, the more radiation it emits. This is the reason you should avoid using so-called radiation shields (the shiny stickers that claim to block radiation); they actually force the phone to transmit at a higher power.
- *Don't Wear Wireless Headsets as Jewelry*: Get it away from your body when not using it!

1. *Do you consistently do any of the above behaviors that affect the body negatively?*
   _____
   _____
   _____

2. *If yes, what adjustments can you make?*
   _____
   _____
   _____

The American diet – high in meat, sugar, fast food and junk food is very acidic, or high on the pH scale. In America, we eat far too many foods that cause the body to be acidic – meat, sugar, alcohol.

Many nutritionists and doctors recommend an 80% alkaline and 20% acidic diet. This translates to eating more of the foods you see on the chart below. A body with a proper pH balance is simply healthier and less prone to disease. And a great way to accomplish this is to stay with one-ingredient foods, and combinations of them.

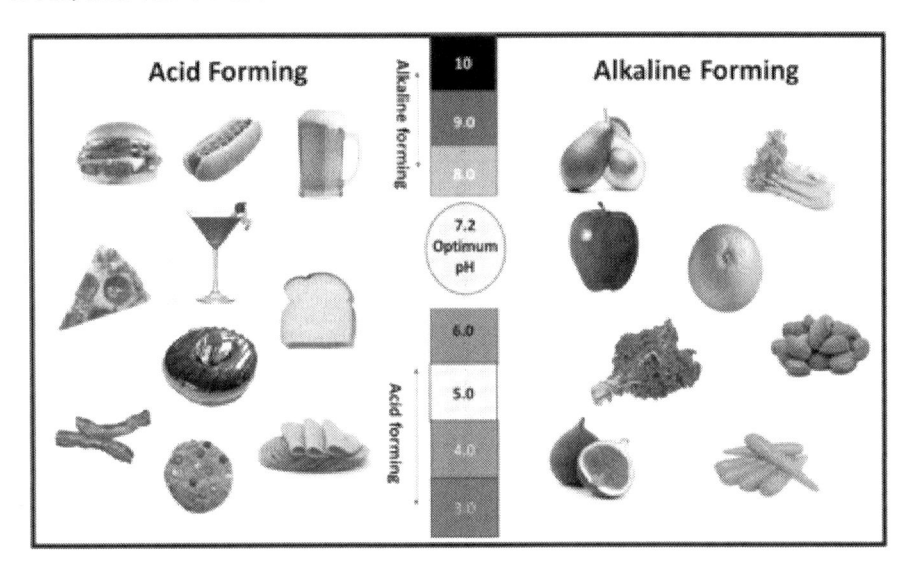

1. As a group, discuss what portion of your diets are on the alkaline side.
_____
_____
_____

Let Food be Thy Medicine and Medicine Thy Food
Hippocrates, 460 BC

Video #6

Topic #1

The Children

I frequently walk in the "climate-controlled" mall in my area. Recently, I noticed another store has opened that caters to larger-sized women and children. That makes a total of six stores – two strictly for larger sizes and four more that have expanded their stock to accommodate our ever-expanding American population.

In 1985, the average American woman wore a size eight. Today, she wears a size 14. Plus-size clothing was worth $17 billion in sales last year (NBC). Is it too much sugar? Too much artificial food? Too much fast food? Too many soft drinks? Or maybe just too much of everything in general?

Maps of Obesity

The obesity trend in America has skyrocketed, as evidenced by the U.S. maps shown on the video. In 1985, 10-15% of Americans were overweight. By 2015, the rate rose to 40%. Three states – Louisiana, Mississippi, West Virginia – are over 40%. "Today, about one in three American kids and teens are overweight or obese. 23.9 million children ages 2 to 19 are overweight or obese." (American Heart Association.)

Obesity is a serious concern because it is associated with poorer mental health, reduced quality of life, and is the leading causes of death in the U.S. It is also associated with diabetes, heart disease, stroke, and some types of cancer. And it's not just the adults. The kids are becoming fatter and fatter.

Parents Outlive Kids

New studies say the above diseases are likely to strike people at younger and younger ages. The study contends that the rapid rise in childhood obesity, if left unchecked, could shorten life spans by as much as five years.

"Obesity is such that this generation of children could be the first basically in the history of the United States to live less healthful and shorter lives than their parents," said Dr. David S. Ludwig, director of the obesity program at *Children's Hospital Boston.*

1. *What could you do in your family, schools, neighborhood or community to help alleviate this problem? Stop buying soft drinks? Shop for foods made from whole grains? Shun unhealthy snacks like doughnuts and candy? Even one small step is a step in the right direction.*

   _____
   _____
   _____

2. *Educating your family on the dangers of eating unhealthy foods and living a sedentary lifestyle will help. What could you do to educate them?*

   _____
   _____
   _____

3. *If you have children, do you see this trend in their friends and classmates?*

   _____
   _____
   _____

Topic #2

Food Deserts

Who would have thought that in America, we would have food deserts? Have you heard of them? Food deserts are areas where whole, unprocessed foods are *not* available. In these areas, the residents don't have cars and there is no supermarket within one mile. They eat foods from local convenience stores. Over 23 million adults and kids live in food deserts (dosomething.org).

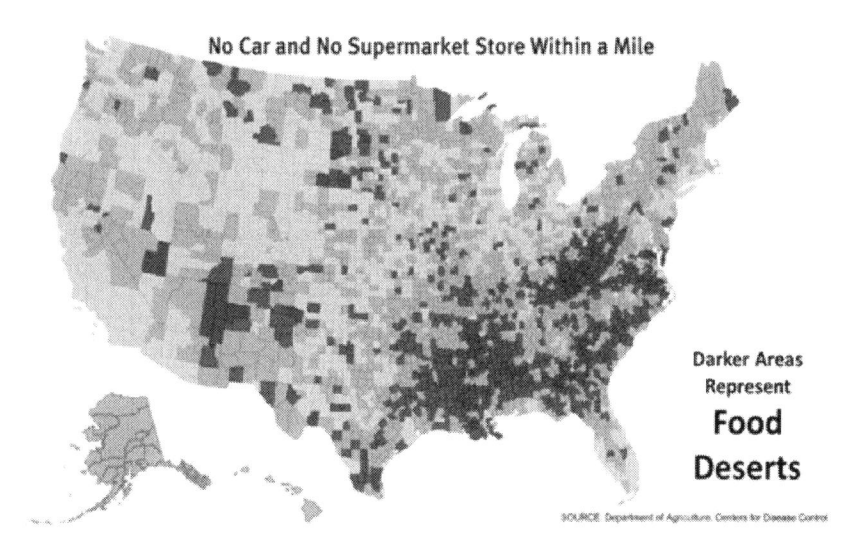

No Car and No Supermarket Store Within a Mile

Darker Areas Represent **Food Deserts**

SOURCE: Department of Agriculture, Centers for Disease Control

1. *Do you think these kids could be fulfilling the suggestion that this generation of children could be the first to live shorter lives than their parents?*
   _____
   _____
   _____

2. *If you lived in a food desert, how would you feed your family in a healthy way?*
   _____
   _____
   _____

3. *Can you think of many healthy foods in a quick mart?*
   _____
   _____
   _____

Moldovan Kids

I was recently on a mission trip to Moldova which is in Eastern Europe. Several of us were there to teach summer school to 150 kids. Lunch generally consisted of the national soup – borscht. It's a thin, vegetable based soup with beets. The kids would place a dollop of sour cream and fresh dill on top. The drink was bottled apple juice, no sugar added. And there was always a plate of sliced bread and fresh tomatoes and cucumbers (every meal).

I watched those kids devour their bread and borscht – with gusto! I couldn't help but wonder – how would American kids – accustomed to hamburgers, fries, sugared drinks and pizza – respond to that lunch? By the way, not one of those kids had an extra pound on their body!

1. *Although American kids might not like Borscht, what are some healthy lunches that you could make for your children to eat?*
   _____
   _____
   _____

2. *What can you do to encourage them to eschew the junk foods and choose the healthy ones?*

   _____
   _____

3. *Occasional slips are inevitable (think holidays), but do you see how a daily lifestyle of unhealthy foods leads to the dismal situation our country is in at this time?*

   _____
   _____

4. *Do your children eat a school lunch? What do they get for school lunch?*

   _____
   _____
   _____

Jamie Oliver Celebrity Chef TV Special

In the fall of 2009, the British celebrity-chef Jamie Oliver arrived in Huntington, West Virginia which was coined "the unhealthiest city in America." Oliver had come to save them, and to film a TV program – "Food Revolution."

Oliver had a difficult time convincing the kitchen help that his was a worthy cause. They did not want to change the way they'd always prepared their foods – commercially prepared selections out of boxes, cans and tubes.

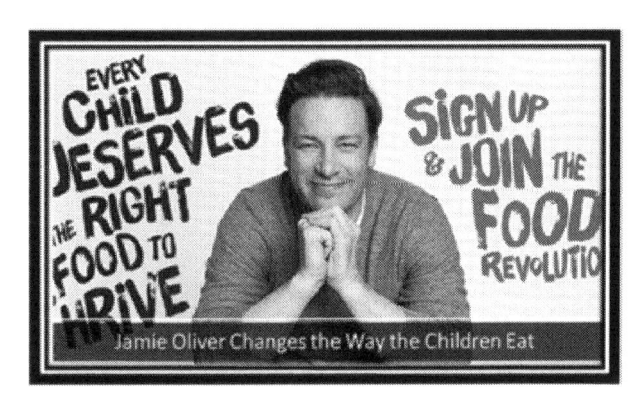

Jamie Oliver Changes the Way the Children Eat

1. *Did you see the special? If you have a chance, go to YouTube where you can view the show.*
   _____
   _____
   _____

2. *It seems to me that the only way we are going to stop the obesity trend in our kids and extend their lives is to help them to be open to trying new things and looking at foods in a new and healthier way. Do you agree?*
   _____
   _____
   _____

3. *Discuss this point in your group.*
   _____
   _____
   _____

Topic #3

Problems with Processed Foods

Microwave Popcorn

More than half of what Americans eat is ultra-processed, and those foods account for 90 percent of U.S. added sugar intake, new research says (the Atlantic). Thousands of our foods in the marketplace are processed, artificial, sugared, nutrient-deficient, fiber-less, enhanced, on and on.

Microwave popcorn is just one example A disease called *bronchiolitis obliterans or popcorn lung* has shown up in people working in microwave popcorn factories (Nat Inst Occ Safety and Health). Diacetyl – the synthetic butter flavor used – vaporizes and becomes toxic when heated. Try making popcorn on the stove or in an air popper.

More Processed Foods

Let's not give all the other food processing techniques a free ride! Consider that:

- **Artificial Sweeteners** with the amino acid aspartame cross the blood-brain barrier to attack your brain cells, creating a toxic cellular overstimulation called *excitotoxicity*, or cell death.

- **Artificial Flavors** could be a blend of hundreds of additives. Strawberry artificial flavor can contain nearly 50 chemical ingredients.
- **Monosodium Glutamate** is an excitotoxin, which means it overexcites your cells to the point of damage or death, causing brain dysfunction.
- **Artificial Colors** give nice color but nine approved food dyes are linked to cancer, hyperactivity and allergies. Red # 40, which is the most widely used dye, was shown to be connected with tumors in mice.
- **High Fructose Corn Syrup** gets shuttled to your liver and reacts like alcohol.
- **Preservatives** lengthen the shelf-life of foods increasing manufacturers' profits, but are linked to cancer, allergic reactions and more.
- **Emulsifiers** keep foods like salad dressing and ice cream from separating (who said oil and water don't mix)?

Boxed Cereals

Popularly advertised kid's cereals are high in sugar, low in nutrition and expensive! Cornell researchers found that cereals marketed to kids are placed half as high on supermarket shelves as adult cereals. The average height for children's cereal boxes is 23 inches versus 48 inches for adult (foodpsychology.cornell.edu).

Natural food stores have excellent tasting and highly nutritious cereals. They are even packaged with labels that kids will like. And they are generally less expensive.

1. *Think about the last time you went to the store with your children. What was their reaction to the cereal aisle? How did they behave if you said "No" to their asking for the "eye level" cereals?*

   _____
   _____
   _____

Healthy Snacks

There are a variety of healthy snack ideas and many are discussed on the video. Popcorn can be made in an air popper or on the stove. Make your own healthy caramel corn by adding honey, molasses and nuts. See the internet on how to make delicious "kale" chips, natural soda, popsicles and frozen yogurt bars.

1. *Please share any healthy snack ideas you have or would like to try.*
   _____
   _____
   _____

Topic #4

Screen Time

The average 2-5-year-old sits in front of a screen 28 hours a week and the average 6-11-year-old increases that amount to 32 hours a week. As most parents know, getting kids away from screens can be a battle. But experts all agree: too much screen time is detrimental to kids. Too much screen time has become epidemic.

Obesity, unhealthy eating habits (from commercials), poor sleep, problems in school, narrowed eye blood vessels, physical problems with hands, fingers and neck (text neck) are all associated with too much of this habit.

Experts recommend keeping all screens outside of bedrooms, restricting time during meals, or using screen time as a reward for reading a book or doing homework (StateFarm.com).

1. *What other ideas can you share with the group of ways to limit screen time?*
   _____
   _____
   _____

Train Up a Child in The Way They Should Go, And When They Are Old, They Will Not Depart from It

Proverbs 22:6

Video #7

Topic #1

Fermenting

Although fermented foods – foods preserved by the action of microorganisms – have become trendy in recent years, the process is not really new, at all. In fact, cultures worldwide have had their fermented "favorites" for centuries.

How Fermenting Works

Fermented foods go through a process of lacto-fermentation. This means that as natural bacteria forms in the fermentation process, the sugar and starches in the food create lactic acid. As the "sitting and steeping" progresses, beneficial enzymes (help break down food), B-vitamins (the anti-stress vitamins) and probiotics (good for gut) are produced – substances for gut health, for fighting allergies and many other conditions.

Keep in mind that canned sauerkraut won't give the same benefits as those "made from scratch" because of the heat applied during canning. Check the internet for recipes, or go to Mercola.com.

1. *Do you have stress? Stomach problems? Discuss why the probiotics, B-vitamins and enzymes are good for those kinds of health issues.*

   _____
   _____
   _____

2. *Is fermenting something you might do?*

   _____
   _____
   _____

Topic #2

Herbs

Now let's move to the topic of herbs. Long before pharmaceuticals, herbs were the medicine of choice. In the 5th century B.C., Hippocrates, the famous Greek physician, listed approximately 400 herbs in common use. And Native Americans introduced the colonists to plants and herbs such as Black Cohosh, which is still used today for relieving menstrual cramps and menopause symptoms.

Currently, the *World Health Organization* estimates that 80% of people rely on herbal medicines for some part of their primary healthcare. In fact, 70% of German physicians prescribe plant-based medicines.

The Multi-Faceted Benefits of Herbs

There is an herb for every condition imaginable. Herbs can relax spasms, ease pain, alleviate migraines, arrest blood flow, relieve constipation, reduce stress…the list is endless. I discussed several on the video. Here, we will look at several additional herbs and their specific uses and health benefits. Let's start with my top favorite five! (Note: Only take herbs according to the instructions on the bottle and never take any without your doctor's consent if you are pregnant, nursing or trying to get pregnant.)

Favorite Herbs

I've always had herbs in the medicine cabinet or kitchen cupboard. When one of my kids ran in with a skinned knee or bee sting, it was an herb I'd grab. These are my top five favorites because I've seen them work firsthand many times – almost miraculously!

#1 Ginger

Ginger is a natural stomach calmative as reported in many studies, and as witnessed by Danish sailors at high sea. Those given ginger capsules had a greatly reduced chance of seasickness and vomiting!

If you can't stop dry heaving from a migraine, try ginger tea, or a little straight powdered ginger in water. When my kids were little and driving me "up the wall" with a nagging, dry cough, I'd make this formula (and still do):

Cough Stopper

1 teaspoon ginger
1 teaspoon cayenne
1 Tablespoon apple cider vinegar
1 Tablespoon honey
1 Tablespoon hot water to dissolve

Mix together. Take as needed to ease a dry cough

1. *Can you think of any other ways to use ginger? Look on the internet and bring some recipes in to the next meeting.*

   _____
   _____
   _____

#2 Cayenne

If you've ever cut yourself chopping vegetables or shaving, think cayenne. You can sprinkle it directly onto the wound, or make a thick solution by mixing it with a little water. Then, saturate a piece of cloth and place it over the cut. I sprinkle the cut with common grocery store variety cayenne. It works every time!

1. *Think of other uses for cayenne and share them with the group.*
   _____
   _____
   _____

#3 Comfrey

This pesky weed might be growing right in your backyard. Comfrey is my very favorite herb. It is widely known as one of nature's greatest medicinal herbals. Comfrey has an ingredient called "allantoin," thought responsible for its healing benefits. I saw a diabetic foot ulcer heal with a comfrey poultice. When doctors could not seem to clear the sore, comfrey did the trick!

Years ago, my oldest son sat down on his bike, not knowing it was still scalding hot where his newspaper carrier had been welded in place. He incurred a quarter size burn on his inner thigh. Ouch!

I immediately made a comfrey poultice, which is like a giant bandage, and placed it on the burn. We watched that burn form a perfect circular scab – like he'd taken a pen and drawn around the outer edges – in just a couple hours. It fell off a few days later with no scar.

To make a poultice: take cheese cloth or other similar material and place some finely chopped comfrey (root and leaves) in the center. Fold like a bandage. Then, wet it with some warm water and massage it to activate the ingredients. Only use comfrey externally. There are comfrey ointments in natural food stores. Keep it on hand!

1. *Have you ever made a poultice?*
   _____
   _____
   _____

#4 Aloe Vera

The gel inside the leaves of the Aloe plant can be used externally to treat minor burns, sunburn, cuts, scrapes and poison ivy. It removes plaque from teeth, and is available as a toothpaste. Many people use it to reduce acne and treat other skin problems.

I've always been told that the wrinkles of aging – caused from a lack of collagen – can't be reversed. Yet, the conclusion of a study reported in the *Annals of Dermatology* was that facial wrinkles are reduced remarkably with Aloe Vera.

In the above study, Aloe was taken as a supplement (around 2000 mg, daily). Consider buying prepared aloe gel (pure, with nothing artificial) and rubbing in on the wrinkled areas. Also keep an aloe plant in your home and harvest the "goo" from the broken off leaves.

1. *The video mentioned another use for Aloe Vera, what was it?*
   _____
   _____
   _____

#5 – Nettles

This stinging weed grows wild and was another "pest" in my backyard that we used for making tea. We would gather the leaves and root, and make tea at the onset of a cold. It is also good for your respiratory system, sinuses, to promote lactation and ease gingivitis. One if its most popular uses is to treat urinary problems during the early stages of an enlarged prostate – called benign prostatic hyperplasia (Univ. Maryland Med. Ctr.).

More Herbs

Far beyond my "favorite five," there are hundreds of herbs – from every corner of the earth – that can be made into teas, infusions, poultices, encapsulated, compresses, baths, ointments, syrups…and more. Here are several.

Chasteberry – Chasteberry is a tree that produces red-black berries. It's been used extensively for female problems such as **PMS** and cramping. The berry normalizes the ratio of progesterone to estrogen, which eases monthly cycle issues. In one study of premenstrual women, 90 percent of those who took the herb reported a reduction in PMS symptoms (Textbook of Natural Medicine).

Cinnamon – Cinnamon helps **lower blood sugar** levels and improves sensitivity to the hormone insulin (Diabetes Obese Metab. 2009). Common "kitchen" cinnamon is hard on the liver, in large quantities. *Use a supplement with cinnamomum verum or cinnamomum cassi.*

> 1. Are you starting to see how you can incorporate herbs into your life in a positive manner, even if you are simply adding them to your meals? Turmeric in stir fry; cinnamon in oatmeal; thyme in homemade soup; ginger in muffins; cayenne sprinkled of various foods. What other ideas do you have?
>
> _____
> _____
> _____

Hawthorne Berry – Hawthorn is used to **support the heart**, lower blood pressure and smooth arrhythmia. It is rich in healthy antioxidants. In one study, when volunteers took 900 milligrams per day of hawthorn extract for two months, it was as effective as low doses of a popular heart medication (Eur J Heart Fail 2009).

Thyme – Thyme has the volatile oil *thymol*, a potent **antiseptic** that kills intestinal microorganisms. It's good for easing mouth sores. Make a poultice of crushed fresh thyme, and apply the poultice to the neck area to reduce throat infections. To relieve congestion, asthma, and whooping cough, try a teaspoonful of thyme extract mixed with an equal amount of honey. Buy online or at a natural food store.

Turmeric – Called by some a miracle herb, turmeric is known to promote healthy aging of cells. While turmeric is a spice used in cooking, the powerful active ingredient within – **curcumin** – is extracted and used as a supplement to reduce inflammation. Inflammation is linked to *all diseases*. It is effective for heart disease and brain conditions like Alzheimer's (Adv Exp Med Bio 2007).

1. *Do you have any favorite herbs? Share with the group what they are and how you use them.*
   _____
   _____
   _____

These are just a few examples of herbs, and how they can be used. But don't stop with the ones we've talked about. If your curiosity has been stirred, become a student.

There's a wealth to knowledge about herbs and how you can take advantage of their health-giving benefits. You never know when you might step onto an elevator and hear someone say, "I have a terrible migraine." And you'll have the chance to respond, "Have you heard about Feverfew?"

I Have Given You Every Herb Bearing Seed Which is on the Face of All the Earth, and Every Tree, in the Which is the Fruit of a Tree Yielding Seed: to you it Shall be for Meat

Genesis 1:29

Video #8

Topic #1

VITAL VITAMINS

It was Dr. Cashmere Funk who coined the word "vitamin" in 1910, when he noticed cultures worldwide got diseases from dietary deficiencies. For example, he found that when "rice-eating" cultures began refining their rice – polishing it to remove the bran and fiber – they got the disease *beriberi* (a lack of thiamine or B1).

Vitamin B1 is needed for a healthy brain and nervous system, as well as for healthy skin, hair, eyes, and liver. When rice is refined (polished), roughly 80% of the B1 and other vitamins are removed. Brown rice contains all the original nutrients because it is a *whole food* – the way nature made it. *And so, food processing and refining rears its ugly head again!*

1. *Most of the time, do you eat brown or white rice?*
   _____
   _____

2. *Can you see how a lifetime of eating processed foods will reduce or eliminate your nutritional stores?*
   _____
   _____

Vitamin A

Vitamin A is needed for healthy skin and respiratory tract. Vitamin A is important for any body part that opens to the outside (ears, mouth, lungs, colon). Sweet potatoes, carrots, spinach, peppers and tomatoes are examples of Vitamin A-containing vegetables. In some studies, adequate vitamin A has been shown to significantly reduced colon cancer risks.

1. *What could you do to increase your family's intake of Vitamin A vegetables? Sweet potato chunks in smoothies? Spinach and peppers in an omelet?*
   _____
   _____
   _____

The B Vitamin Complex

I call the B's the *stress vitamins*. There are many of them but as a group, they are called the B Complex vitamins. One study showed that the B vitamins slowed brain shrinkage in regions severely impacted by Alzheimer's (Nat Academy of Sciences). Good food choices are legumes, lean meats, whole grains, mushrooms, sunflower seeds, tuna, potatoes, cottage cheese, avocados, broccoli, green beans, spinach, fish and bananas.

1. *Since many of us are under stress, can you see the benefit of eating or supplementing with Vitamin B?*
   _____
   _____
   _____

2. *How could you increase your intake of Vitamin B foods?*
   _____
   _____
   _____

3. On the list of B-vitamin-rich foods, do you see anything processed?

_____
_____
_____

Vitamin C

We all know that vitamin C is good for colds and the flu, but it's also a great antioxidant, which means it stops oxidation (like rusting) in your body. In just one study, cholesterol fell in people taking one added gram of vitamin C a day *(the Lancet)*. In other studies, adequate C improved the sperm count in men. It's in Brussel sprouts, broccoli, strawberries, pineapple, red peppers and kale.

1. Can you think of a way to get more Vitamin C-rich fruits and vegetables into your diet? Check out forksoverknives.com. It has many recipes for blender drinks which kids love, and which are high in Vitamin C.

_____
_____
_____

2. Which snack would have the most vitamin C: Diced fresh strawberries and pineapple OR a candy bar and a soft drink?

_____
_____
_____

Vitamin D

Vitamin D: Get sunshine and eat nuts, whole grains, eggs and fish. Multifunctional Vitamin D is protective against many diseases like cancer, diabetes and multiple sclerosis. It's been shown to decrease the chance of developing heart disease when you have adequate amounts (Circulation Journal).

1. Which breakfast do you think would provide the most vitamin D: (1) walnuts, oatmeal and almond milk which is eaten while sitting in the morning sun OR (2) sugared-cereal with added sugar and a doughnut eaten while sitting in a dark basement?
   _____
   _____
   _____

Vitamin E

Vitamin E is an antioxidant vitamin. A simple explanation: much the same way an automobile rusts over time when exposed to water and air, internal rusting (oxidation) results in your body from not getting enough vitamin E. It's found in nuts, seeds, avocados, healthy oils (not hydrogenated), dark leafy greens and papaya.

1. Which snack would provide the most vitamin E? (1) guacamole (2) sugar cookies (3) jam on white bread
   _____
   _____

2. Are you starting to see that refined and processed foods are deficient in ALL the vitamins?
   _____
   _____
   _____

Topic #2

Mighty Minerals

The processed, packaged, refined, sugared foods that many people live on today are extremely deficient in minerals. You receive minerals by eating plants that absorb them from the earth, or by eating meat from animals, which graze on plants. Here are just a few of the many minerals:

- **Zinc**: Assists in wound healing. Sign of deficiency is reduced sense of smell and taste. Foods include kidney beans, flaxseeds, oysters and pumpkin seeds. When I worked for Jonathan Wright MD, he had a pre-surgery formula that he recommended to patients: Two weeks prior to surgery take 1,000 mg twice daily vitamin C (promotes healing of connective tissue); 30 mg once daily of zinc picolinate (wound healer); vitamin B12 and folic acid as suggested on bottle.
- **Selenium:** May help prevent coronary heart disease. Fights inflammation. Foods include Brazil nuts, yellowfin tuna, halibut, sardines, grass-fed beef.
- **Magnesium:** In one study on 30,000 males, they were shown to have a lower risk of hypertension with a magnesium-rich diet (Harvard School of Public Health). Magnesium is a relaxant. When I worked at the Tahoma Clinic, if a person came in with a migraine, they'd likely

be sent to the IV room for a magnesium IV. Foods include kidney beans, brown rice and avocados.
- **Calcium:** Strong bones, healthy heart, calm nerves. You don't have to drink milk to get calcium. You can also get it in kale, sardines, broccoli and watercress.

1. *Discuss a mineral rich dinner. What would it consist of?*
   _____
   _____
   _____

2. *How can you increase the amount of minerals your family is ingesting? By simply starting to eat whole, natural foods, most of the time?*
   _____
   _____
   _____

Topic #3

Reading Your Body Like a Book

Taken from *Library of Food and Vitamin Cures* by Jonathan V. Wright MD

In my years of working with Jonathan Wright MD, at the renowned Tahoma Clinic in Washington state, I learned why and how to look for signs that could point to nutritional deficiencies. Here's how it works.

Your skin, fingernails, hair and other body parts can point to larger health problems. They can be good indicators of where you might benefit from boosting your nutritional intake – where your body could use a little "help." If you find any signs that you'd like to have checked out, it's a good idea to consult with a doctor skilled in nutritional medicine for help determining what supplement or dietary changes would be beneficial (refer to his book above for more information).

Teenage Acne: Get off refined sugar and soft drinks; add zinc-rich foods to the diet. These include pumpkin seeds, mushrooms, spinach, chicken and garbanzo beans; add essential fatty acids (good fats) like raw sunflower and pumpkin seeds, nuts and olive oil; check for food sensitivities.

Varicose Veins: Go heavy on flavonoids – the substance that gives foods like blueberries, citrus fruits, tomatoes and kale their bright colors. Stay hydrated;

eat fiber-rich foods to reduce downward pressure from constipation; eat magnesium-rich foods to relax veins and arteries.

1. Does anyone remember some magnesium-rich foods?
   _____
   _____
   _____

Calloused and Cracked Feet: Increase essential fatty acids with raw nuts and seeds; flaxseed oil is a good choice – a Tablespoon a day for three months.

Bleeding Gums: Think supplemental Coenzyme Q10. A folate (folic acid/folate is a B vitamin) mouthwash may be beneficial.

Cracks Behind the Ears: Fish oil supplementation along with more essential fatty acids. And don't forget the B vitamins. They are in all your dark leafy greens. Standard grocery store bottled oils are rancid before you even open them because of the extremely high heat applied in processing. Switch to high quality olive oil or grapeseed oil that are "cold-processed." Also, try sprinkling flaxseeds on your cereals or salads. (Don't swallow them whole; chew them well).

1. Do you buy standard bottled oils – the ones that line the grocery shelves?
   _____
   _____
   _____

2. Do you think you might shun them in favor of healthier "cold-processed" choices?
   _____
   _____
   _____

Scalloped Tongue: This is just one of many signs that show on the tongue. While this can be from pressure against the teeth, also think food sensitivities (swelling is a sensitivity reaction). Go to HealthTreasureChest.com for a home test sample, or for a blood test (ALCAT). See Dr. Wright's book for more signs that show on the tongue.

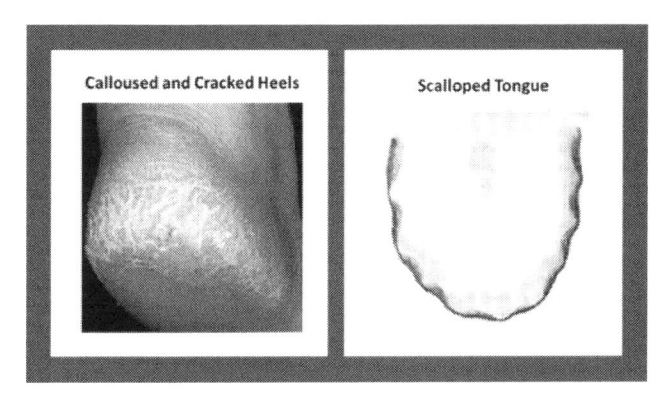

Canker Sores: Can be from food sensitivities. Watch for foods that trigger sores, then eliminate from diet. One of my sons gets bad canker sores from pineapple. There is an herbal "canker sore formula" on my website (products & services tab).

Dry Flaky Scalp: This is usually caused by too much refined sugar and not enough fatty acids.

Dark Circles Under Eyes: Ever see kids who look like their eyes are bruised? Think food sensitivities, especially in kids. According to Jonathan Wright MD, "Nearly all children diagnosed with "hyperactivity" have allergies and sensitivities, especially food allergies. Try eliminating dairy and refined sugars and observe the results."

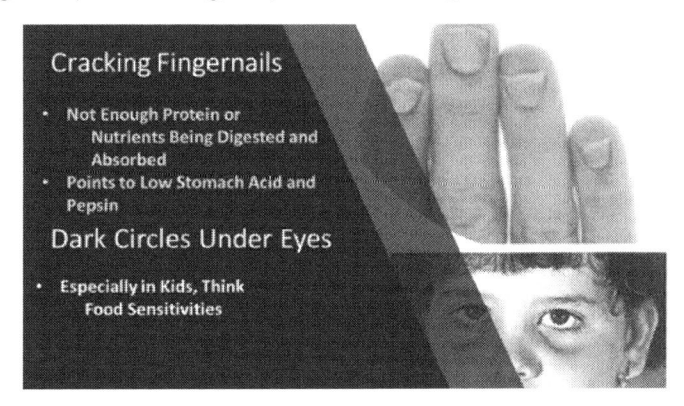

- **White Spots on Fingernails:** Could be a zinc deficiency; go for the zinc-rich foods such as: spinach, kidney beans, flax seeds, pumpkin seeds.

Take the Telomere Test to Find Out the State of Your Health

If you want to know how healthy you are, consider taking the *Telomere Test for Aging*. It's a simple blood test that helps determine your susceptibility to chronic disease. If interested, check out internet or go to my website for information and ordering (*Products & Services on Video tab*).

Topic #4

NATURAL CLEANING SOLUTIONS

Have you ever paid attention to the strong, toxic smells radiating out of the cleaning aisle in the grocery store? Make-at-home natural cleaning solutions do an excellent job, are nontoxic, cost very little and don't leave behind chemical smells. You can also make them right in your kitchen and save lots of money.

Here are the ingredients you'll need: baking soda, white vinegar, hydrogen peroxide, Borax soap, glycerin, lemon juice, liquid soap, oxy-clean, corn starch, alcohol and essential oils, if desired. All the recipes are at HealthTreasureChest.com (products & services tab). So, mix away and protect yourself and your family from toxic, smelly chemicals.

1. *Look on the website and evaluate the recipes there for cleaners.*
   _____
   _____
   _____

Kathryn Parslow PhD, CCN

The Food You Eat Can be the Safest and the Most Powerful Form of Medicine or the Slowest Form of Poison
Ann Wigmore, Wheatgrass Movement

Video #9

Topic #1

FOODS THAT HEAL

When you are eating whole, natural, unadulterated foods – not the artificial selections in packages, boxes and cans – you can benefit from their healing powers. That's right. Foods can heal!

Here are just a few examples of their therapeutic powers. But don't stop here. Take advantage of all the earth offers. If you'll just stay away from the junk foods provided by the processed food industry, you can reap remarkable rejuvenation and healing benefits.

- **Brazil Nuts:** The #1 richest source of the mineral selenium, Brazil nuts stave off **depression**. Researchers at *Swansea University* in the United Kingdom found that just 100-micrograms of selenium provided the mood-changing benefits. Just a few Brazil nuts a week are all you need – (you can overdo with Brazil nuts).
- **Cabbage:** Anti-cancer; in studies, eating cabbage more than once a week cut men's **colon cancer** risks by 66%.
- **Cherries:** A new *Boston University* study on hundreds of patients confirmed that eating three servings of cherries – about 1½ cups before a full-on **gout** attack – was the magic number for prevention. Cherries are known to reduce uric acid levels.

- **Cloves:** Long used to relieve the pain of **toothache,** its main ingredient – eugenol – is anti-inflammatory and will reduce inflammation in the body.
- **Figs:** Figs contain a substance known as benzaldehyde, a flavonoid that has powerful **anti-cancer** effects (Plant Foods Hum Nutr).

1. *Figs are not commonly eaten. 2 Kings 20:7 says of Hezekiah, "Prepare a poultice of figs. They did so and applied it to the boil, and he recovered." Besides eating them raw, do you have any recipes using figs you can share with the group?*

_____

_____

_____

- **Pineapple:** Animals deficient in manganese develop severe **osteoporosis,** according to a study from the *University of Texas*. Pineapple is a good source.
- **Garlic:** People have known since time immemorial that garlic is a healer. In just one study of many, people who ate garlic had a 35 percent lower risk of getting **colon cancer** *(Univ. Maryland Medical Center)*.
- **Ginger:** Danish sailors sailing at high sea who took one gram of ginger had a 38% reduction in **vomiting and nausea,** as compared to those who did not take ginger.
- **Mixed Raw Nuts**: In a study of over 30,000 Seventh Day Adventists (who eat an extremely healthy diet), those eating raw and uncooked nuts five times a week cut their heart attack risks in half.

2. *From just this small sampling attesting to the benefits of eating whole foods, do you think it would be beneficial to incorporate them into your diet?*

_____

_____

_____

3. *Discuss – as a group – how your health might improve if you ate foods like these – day after day, year after year.*

   _____
   _____
   _____

4. *What can you do to begin to add more whole foods to your family's diet?*

   _____
   _____
   _____

Note: You'll hear on the video my 90-10 rule. This means, 90 percent of the time, eat whole, one-ingredient foods or combinations of them. And the other 10 percent? Enjoy some of your favorite foods that might not appear on the "healthiest" list. Let's call it "recreational" eating.

Topic #2

The Nutrition Researchers Who Went Before

Preserving the history of nutrition for future generations has always been a priority of mine. It was in 460 BC that Hippocrates, considered the father of medicine said, "Let your food be your medicine and your medicine be your food."

Down through the generations, others have followed the "Hippocratic Oath," believing that it matters what we eat. Here are six of them I consider *nutritional giants*:

Weston A. Price DDS (1847-1998)

Weston A. Price was a dentist. He left his practice at age 50 and travelled with his wife to every continent for a 10-year period. His quest: to study teeth and jaws. What he discovered was that when people stayed with their native diet (which was extremely varied worldwide, with some vegetarians and some not), they were healthy, generation after generation.

But when they began eating what he called the "foods of commerce" (military PX's, etc.), they began to lose their strong facial structure and their teeth started to decay and deform. There were also other deformities.

His book, *Nutrition and Physical Degeneration* is considered one of the most important works of the 20th century (view his video on YouTube; consider getting it into your kid's schools).

1. Discuss the benefits of his research and how it affects you?
   _____
   _____
   _____

Francis Pottenger MD (1901-1967)

Francis Pottenger was a California doctor who was researching adrenal gland extract. Cats were used in the study. When locals got wind, cats mysteriously began to appear on the sanitorium porch. In the beginning, he fed his cats left over "human-food" scraps from the sanitorium meal trays.

But, as more cats appeared and cat-food supplies diminished, he asked the local butcher for raw meat scraps. Thus, began the 10-year study by Dr. Pottenger.

He conceived of an experiment in which one group of cats received only raw milk and raw meat (traditional cat diet), while other groups received cooked meat, pasteurized milk, sweetened condensed milk and scrapes left over from the patient's plates.

The cats on the raw meat and raw milk diet – a normal cat diet – were healthy, generation after generation. But the cats on deficient diets developed "facial deformities" narrowed faces and frail bones. They had parasites, multiple diseases and difficult pregnancies. Female cats became aggressive while males became docile. After just three generations, young animals died before reaching adulthood and reproduction ceased. His book is, *Pottenger's Cats: A Study in Nutrition.*

1. *Many people say this 1940's diet was inhumane. But there is a lesson to be learned: healthy kids need whole, unrefined, un-sugared foods. Yet, many*

people feed their children deficient foods just like the sick cats received. Do you have any thoughts or comments on this?

_____
_____
_____

Otto Schaeffer MD 1919-2009

Otto Schaeffer MD was the physician to the *Inuit* people of Canada. He found that they were healthy – generation after generation – if they stayed with their native diets. However, when the military came in and they began working at the PX and eating processed foods, their health rapidly began to deteriorate, just like Pottenger's cats and Dr. Price's cultures. It's all recorded in his book, *Sunrise Over Pangnirtung*.

1. *What does this research tell us about what we eat?*

_____
_____
_____

Elizabeth Baker 1913-2007

Elizabeth Baker was sick most of her life. At 59 – at deaths door – she decided to get well. And get well she did! So, she began juicing, drinking mega-doses of wheatgrass and eating all raw foods (nuts, seeds, fruits and vegetables; not raw meat).

It took two years, but she did get well and went on to write eight books on raw foods. She taught thousands the value of eating a healthy diet with lots of raw food. She was considered the "raw food" lady of the land.

Elizabeth Baker – my dear friend and mentor – willed me her story of recovery. It was written on old, yellowed typing paper. I felt the information so valuable, that I included in my book, *How to Survive the American High-Tech Diet* (available at HealthTreasureChest.com).

How to Survive the American High-Tech Diet

1. *What choices can you make to include more raw vegetables, fruits, nuts and seeds into your diet?*

   _____
   _____
   _____

Ann Wigmore 1909-1993

Ann Wigmore was scheduled to have her feet amputated from a car accident. She refused. Instead, remembering her grandmother saying, "instinct-guided creatures left to themselves do not make mistakes," she sat in her backyard all summer and chewed grass.

In time, her feet healed completely and she went on to run the Boston Marathon. She is the originator of wheatgrass, the healthy beverage craze available in health food stores.

- *Have you ever tried wheatgrass? To make it at home requires a special grinding juicer.*
- *Many juice bars provide shots of wheatgrass. Give it a try!*

Denis Burkitt MD 1911-1993

Denis Burkitt MD was considered "the fiber doctor." He travelled Africa studying the dietary habits of native Africans and found that they don't get the diseases of his native Englishman such as cancer, heart disease, colon disease etc.

He attributed their "wellness" to their native high-fiber diet which caused food to move through their bodies three times as fast as "constipated" Englishmen. They were simply cleaner, internally.

1. *How is your fiber intake?*

   _____
   _____
   _____

2. *How can you increase your intake of fiber-rich whole foods such as raw vegetables like celery and carrots?*
   _____
   _____

3. *Is your bread choice whole grain?*
   _____
   _____

4. *How much fiber is in* white bread, white cake, white cookies, white noodles and pasta, white sugar, breakfast cereals made from white flour and white rice?
   _____
   _____
   _____

How to Survive the American High-Tech Diet

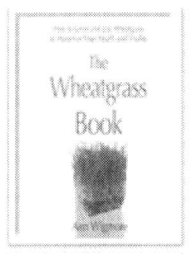

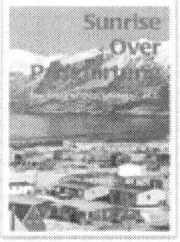

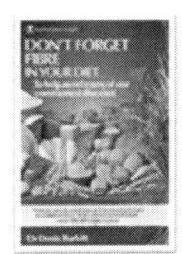

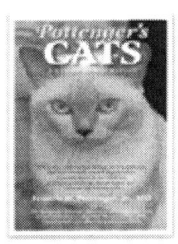

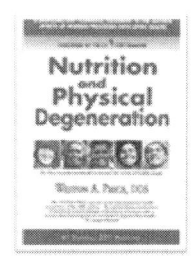

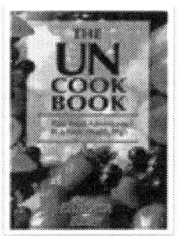

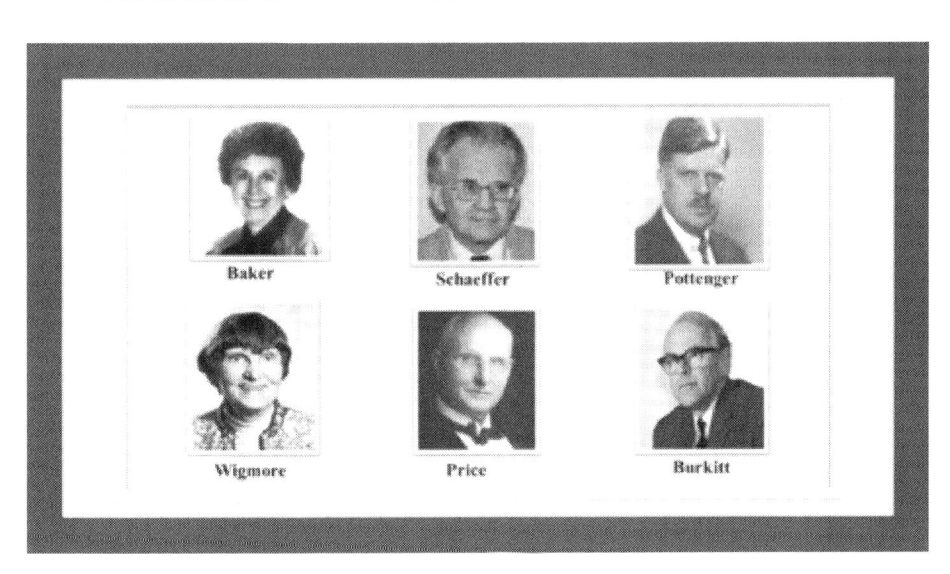

My People Are Destroyed from Lack of Knowledge   Hosea 4:6

Video #10

Topic #1

DETOXIFICATION

Why Detoxify?

I suppose our ancestors didn't need to give body detoxification a second thought. But then, their air didn't have noxious pollutants and their water wasn't contaminated with chlorine, fluoride and arsenic. They didn't sleep on pillows containing polyurethane, or drive in new cars emitting ethylbenzene, formaldehyde, and toluene.

Their foods weren't genetically modified (GMO's), nor were they plied with pesticides. The fact is, the USDA now says 85% of foods tested have pesticide residues. What's a person to do?

Enter body detoxification! Here are just a few ideas you can utilize to begin a detoxification program that will help rid your body of all the modern-day chemicals. There are lots of books on detoxification, if you'd like more information.

Skin Brushing for Detoxifying

Did you know that your skin is classified as an organ – the largest one in your body? It is through the skin that most toxins you eat in or breathe in are eliminated. Dry skin brushing is a simple wellness trick that costs nothing, takes less than five minutes a day, and cleanses your body – inside and out. It works by unclogging pores as dead skin is brushed away. This allows for the excretion of built up internal toxins.

Getting Started with Skin Brushing

To get started, you'll need a natural (not synthetic) bristle brush with a long handle that allows you to reach all areas of your body. Start at your feet and move upward in long sweeping motions, always brushing toward your heart. When brushing shoulders and upper arms, brush downward, toward your heart. Brush several times in each area, overlapping as you go. Take care on more sensitive areas.

Continue brushing for three to five minutes. At this point, you'll want to shower. Many people choose to take intermittent hot and cold showers. You can read about this on the internet.

1. *Have you ever heard of the benefits of skin brushing?*
   _____
   _____
   _____

Dry Saunas

Sauna therapy helps expel toxins through sweating. It also encourages improved blood circulation. In one study, men who used a sauna four to seven times a week had a 66% lower risk of developing dementia, and a 65% lower risk of Alzheimer's, compared to men who used a sauna once a week (Reuters 2017).

And Finnish researchers revealed that men who used the Finnish-style, dry heat sauna seven times per week cut their risk of death from fatal heart problems in half, compared to those who used it only once a week (JAMA).

How to Survive the American High-Tech Diet

George M. Yu MD, teaches a method of detoxifying by taking the B vitamin niacin prior to a sauna session. If you'd like more details on Dr. Yu's protocol, go to Mercola.com.

As another bonus of sauna therapy, many people say their skin is much softer and clearer, and they have a sense of well-being after a session, feeling cleaner, sharper and less toxic.

1. Do you belong to a gym that has a sauna? If yes, how frequently do you use it?

   _____
   _____

2. Discuss the ways in which sweating is beneficial and why you should take advantage of a sauna if you have one available.

   _____
   _____
   _____

Topic # 2

How to Shop for Health

Now, let's move on to what this entire 10-video-series was primarily about: *what we eat*. When you start eating *without needing to read labels* (whole, one-ingredient foods don't need labels), you exponentially increase your chances of having good health. As we've been learning, every time you eat or drink, you are either fueling disease or promoting health.

The less you eat from a box and more from the earth, the greater your chances are of being at your ideal weight and enjoying a disease-free life. The idea is to nourish your body, not just fill an empty stomach. And what you buy at the grocery store will influence that!

Working the Grocery Aisles

Grocery stores are laid out with the healthier foods along the periphery. This is where you'll find produce, meat, seafood, dairy and bulk bins with lots of healthy choices. The packaged, processed junk foods are down the center aisles. Here is where you will find boxed dinners, TV dinners, chips, soda, candy, cookies etc.

1. *What foods do you consistently buy from the periphery of the store?*
   _____
   _____
   _____

2. *Analyze the foods you buy from the center aisles and consider how you could cut down on them or how you could substitute healthier alternatives.*
   _____
   _____
   _____

The Center Aisles

You don't need to totally forsake the center aisles. Look for healthy, natural soups, (avoid the popular brands because of additives); condiments (watch out though – many have lots of sugar or high fructose corn syrup); popcorn (not microwavable), nuts, whole grain pastas and spaghetti sauce.

You can find canned fruits with no sugar, but fresh is always best. Generally, avoid canned vegetables (frozen is better, fresh best). Exceptions are canned beans and tomatoes which are always good to have on hand. Also, canned foods like water chestnuts, enchilada sauce, canned diced chilis – ingredients you might use in recipes – are acceptable.

Choose to buy products in jars instead of cans or plastic bottles, when possible. Many plastic bottles have BPA, a known carcinogen. And, most cans have a plastic lining that is heated when the product is being canned. That lining has BPA unless the can is labeled **BPA free**. The "BPA free" stamp will usually be on the bottom or top of the can.

Generally, avoid frozen dinners including breakfast waffles, microwavable lunch and TV dinners (just turn one over and read the ingredients). Look for frozen popsicles with no sugar added. Check out the sweetener *Stevia* – a healthy choice that is made from a leaf. And only buy organic baby food, or make from scratch.

Regarding baby food, many baby food products have rice as a base. Much of the rice (exception Lundens brand from California) has a high concentration of arsenic. Children's bodies are more susceptible to this poison because they are still developing.

1. *If you pack your lunch and take a microwavable meal, what ideas do you have of what you could pack that would be healthier?*
   _____
   _____
   _____

2. *Remembering the "one-ingredient" rule, what dinners could you make that are simple, quick and don't come from a box or package?*
   _____
   _____
   _____

Go Organic and Additive-Free

Recently, when I was at a supermarket, there was a PA announcement that said, "organic milk on sale." The lady across the aisle from me said out loud, but to herself, "I am so sick of hearing organic, organic, organic! What difference does it make?"

More than 600 chemicals are registered for use in America. This equates to about 16 pounds of chemical pesticides per person, every year. Many were approved prior to EPA testing. These are certainly substances our ancestors did not eat. Shun them when you can.

Natural Food Stores

Most larger grocery stores have natural food sections. Here you will find foods that are far more natural than those in the regular aisles. For example, the cereals will be additive, preservative, and GMO-free, the dairy section will provide products that are organic, and the cleaners and shampoos will be chemical-free. As best you can, eat fresh, whole and additive-free. Organic is a far better choice, any time you can find it.

Some of you may be well on your way to an all-natural, chemical-free, highly nutritious diet. Others may just be getting started, or considering if you even want to change. Remember Jim the trucker? As sick as he was, all he could commit to was "an apple a day." But it was a start!

Final Word

At this point, you've read about Elizabeth Baker – my friend and mentor. Through the years, I taught extensively with her at conferences, even when she was approaching 90. After she would speak, younger women would rush up to the podium and ask, "Elizabeth, what can I <u>take</u> to be healthy?" She would take their hands in hers, look them right in the eyes and say, "My dear, you <u>take</u> the bad out of the diet!"

Do you remember the ladder of achievement? Going from "I won't" to "what is it?" is a huge step. Just make healthy changes as you can and – before you know it – you'll be eating a healthful, lifegiving, disease-preventing diet!

Bon Appetite! *Your partner on the journey*   *Kathryn Parslow*

HealthTreasureChest.com Signature Salad Sprinkle

Use organic and dehydrated fruits; makes 40-one Tablespoon servings. All these ingredients are available on Amazon or natural food stores. Generally, need to be bought in larger quantities. Consider making with friends and sharing cost. Chew well to extract all the healthy benefits!

*¼ cup **Dehydrated Buckwheat Sprouts*** *(powerful flavonoid <u>rutin</u> for heart)*
*¼ cup **Dehydrated Goji Berries*** *(anticancer; pro-eye/hormones/diabetes)*
*¼ cup **Dehydrated Blueberries*** *(antioxidants to support eyes)*

*¼ cup **Dehydrated Cranberries*** *(general wellness + kidney, bladder)*
*¼ cup **Shredded Unsweetened** Coconut (healthy fats maintain lean muscles)*
*¼ cup **Chopped Walnuts*** *(the ultimate brain food)*
*¼ cup **Chopped Almonds*** *(lower cholesterol, heart healthy)*
*¼ cup **Apple Pectin*** *(anti-cancer; used in Chernobyl against radioactivity)*
*¼ cup **Dehydrated Parsley*** *(vitamin K-rich for bones)*

Mix all together and store in airtight container. Use as desired as a salad sprinkle. Keep nuts in refrigerator/freezer until ready to use because they can go rancid due to oil content. If you can't find an item, make without. Sprouted, dehydrated buckwheat available on Amazon (Sun & Seed Organic Sprouted and Raw Buckwheat; make sure to buy sprouted because the unsprouted seed is too hard to chew).

Made in the USA
Lexington, KY
11 October 2017